RESTLESS IN SLEEP COUNTRY

RESTLESS IN SLEEP COUNTRY

Imagination and the Cultural Politics of Sleep

PAUL HUEBENER

MCGILL-QUEEN'S UNIVERSITY PRESS
Montreal & Kingston • London • Chicago

ISBN 978-0-2280-2038-7 (cloth)
ISBN 978-0-2280-2039-4 (paper)
ISBN 978-0-2280-2040-0 (ePDF)
ISBN 978-0-2280-2041-7 (ePUB)

Legal deposit first quarter 2024
Bibliothèque nationale du Québec

Printed in Canada on acid-free paper that is 100% ancient forest free (100% post-consumer recycled), processed chlorine free

This book has been published with the help of a grant from the Canadian Federation for the Humanities and Social Sciences, through the Awards to Scholarly Publications Program, using funds provided by the Social Sciences and Humanities Research Council of Canada.

Funded by the Government of Canada | Financé par le gouvernement du Canada | Canada
Canada Council for the Arts | Conseil des arts du Canada

We acknowledge the support of the Canada Council for the Arts.
Nous remercions le Conseil des arts du Canada de son soutien.

McGill-Queen's University Press in Montreal is on land which long served as a site of meeting and exchange amongst Indigenous Peoples, including the Haudenosaunee and Anishinabeg nations. In Kingston it is situated on the territory of the Haudenosaunee and Anishinaabek. We acknowledge and thank the diverse Indigenous Peoples whose footsteps have marked these territories on which peoples of the world now gather.

LIBRARY AND ARCHIVES CANADA CATALOGUING IN PUBLICATION

Title: Restless in sleep country : imagination and the cultural politics of sleep / Paul Huebener.
Names: Huebener, Paul, author.
Description: Includes bibliographical references and index.
Identifiers: Canadiana (print) 20240287045 | Canadiana (ebook) 20240287061 | ISBN 9780228020394 (paper) | ISBN 9780228020387 (cloth) | ISBN 9780228020400 (ePDF) | ISBN 9780228020417 (ePUB)
Subjects: LCSH: Sleep—Social aspects—Canada. | LCSH: Sleep—Political aspects—Canada. | LCSH: Sleep in literature.
Classification: LCC GT3000.4.C3 H84 2024 | DDC 392.3—dc23

This book is for my dad, Bruce Huebener, who always looks forward to reading my manuscripts. It is also for Carrie Young and the staff at Grey Nuns Community Hospital in Edmonton, who brought Dad back from the brink of Covid-19 during the Delta wave in 2021.

CONTENTS

FIGURES

ACKNOWLEDGMENTS

This book has benefited from the kind support and expertise of many people. First, I thank Niki Boyd for her endless generosity and thoughtfulness, for pointing me toward many articles on sleep, for contemplating the hacking of Wi-Fi-connected mattresses, and for agreeing to include some of our personal family stories in the book. Niki has witnessed my many failures as a sleeper, and when I told her that I wanted to write a book about sleep, she said, "I thought you're supposed to write about what you know." Thank you, Niki, for these inspiring words and for making me laugh.

Many thanks to my incredible editor, Kyla Madden, and to everyone at McGill-Queen's University Press who worked so hard to bring this book to life. Lesley Trites and Lisa Aitken handled many production details, David Drummond created the wonderful cover art, Robert Lewis's copy editing improved the manuscript significantly, and Stephen Ullstrom compiled the index with great skill. Thank you to Kathleen Fraser, Jonathan Crago, and Kyla for proposing a book title that improved on my working title. Thanks as well to Kyla, Jonathan, and Mark Abley for kindly inviting me to return to McGill-Queen's after the press published my first book back in 2015.

I am grateful to Bruce Huebener for reviewing a full draft of the manuscript and for offering nearly two hundred thoughtful comments that led to many useful additions and edits. I thank Julie Stewart and Chris Spencer for agreeing to let me include a story about our shared experience during the Alberta floods of 2013, Ben Lefebvre for advice on publishing, and Pamela Banting for frequent conversation and support throughout this project.

My thanks to Shepherd Steiner for inviting me to give a public lecture for the journal *Mosaic* as part of its Relative Time/Little Time series in 2022, hosted in collaboration with Bik Van der Pol, and to Sabrina Mark, Piu Chowdhury, and Timothy Brown for their work in orchestrating this event. Thank you to Aleksandra Kaminska, Alanna Thain, Charlène Auré, Marianne Cloutier, and the other members of the Sociability of Sleep research group for inviting me to speak at their Sleep Salon event series in 2023. Many thanks to Amanda Farnel and the rest of the program team at the Saskatchewan Festival of Words for inviting me to speak at their event in 2022 and, after I withdrew due to illness, for doubling down on their generosity by reinviting me in 2023. I am grateful to Diletta De Cristofaro, principle investigator of the Writing the Sleep Crisis research group, for her outstanding work in building a community of scholars in critical sleep studies, for directing me toward important sources, and for inviting me to take part in the Sleep and Digital Health conference in 2022. Many thanks as well to the organizers of other conferences where I had the chance to share my work in progress and to hear feedback from colleagues, including the 2020 and 2022 conferences of the Association for Literature, Environment, and Culture in Canada (ALECC), the Athabasca University Faculty of Humanities and Social Sciences Research Seminar and Speaker series in 2021, and the Material Life of Time: The Second International Temporal Belongings Conference in 2021. Thanks to Diletta and the Popular Culture Association for including me in their 2022 conference program and for their gracious understanding when I had to withdraw due to Covid-19. I also thank the community of ALECC members, many of whom responded to my list-serv query about representations of sleep in Canada. ALECC members have been a source of inspiration and support throughout my career.

I am grateful to Cressida Heyes and Nariya Khasanova for sharing their sleep studies bibliography with me, and I thank Michael Greaney, Hilary Hinds, and Garrett Sullivan for developing the useful sleep studies resources previously hosted on their website. I also thank Susie O'Brien for inspiring me to develop assignments that take students beyond the classroom. I am grateful to Athabasca University for enabling my research, and I thank my colleagues there, past and present, who have so thoughtfully supported my sabbatical time and other research leaves, particularly Angie Abdou, Jolene Armstrong, Manijeh Mannani, Marian Allen, Mark McCutcheon, Michael Brisbois, Romita Choudhury, Shawna Cunningham, Sonia Atwal, Veronica Thompson, and Vina Tirven-Gadum.

Many friends and colleagues thoughtfully recommended particular books and other works to me. Thank you to Adam Dickinson, Alec Follett, Ben Lefebvre, Brian Bartlett, Carolyn Veldstra, Colleen Court, Conrad Scott, Dana Mount, David R. Anderson, David Eso, Don McKay, Erin Aspenlieder, Jason Wiens, Jeffery Donaldson, Jenny Kerber, Jessica Barr, Judy Wajcman, Julie Huff, Kate McKenzie, Katja Lee, Kelly Shepherd, Leah Van Dyke, Lisa

Szabo-Jones, Lorraine York, Marilyn Osborne, Mark McCutcheon, Marlene Creates, Matthew Zantingh, Melanie Dennis Unrau, Pam Chamberlain, Rhona McAdam, Simon Orpana, and Trish Audette-Longo.

This book includes discussions of works by Indigenous authors and artists. As a white member of the settler society in Canada, I cannot speak on behalf of Indigenous Peoples, and I have no claim to Indigenous cultural property. As a scholar who wishes to develop an understanding of cultural concerns in Canada, I hope to recognize and engage with the work of Indigenous Peoples, to account for the ongoing consequences of colonization, and to encourage others to read and learn from Indigenous literatures. I have tried to approach this process in accordance with Gregory Younging's advice in his book *Elements of Indigenous Style*. In naming Indigenous Peoples, I have drawn primarily from the self-identifications of the writers I refer to, with additional assistance from the Canadian Association of University Teachers' *Guide to Acknowledging First Peoples and Traditional Territory*. In discussing works of Indigenous literatures alongside works of Canadian literature, I recognize that, as Younging notes, "Indigenous Literatures are their own canon and not a subgroup of CanLit."[1] In light of the fact that Younging's guidelines are meant to be part of an ongoing conversation, and in discussion with McGill-Queen's about best practices for capitalization, I have tried to capitalize terms when necessary in order to indicate specificity while also being mindful of the fact that minimal capitalization is helpful for readability. When referring to insights belonging to Indigenous Traditional Knowledge, I have tried to rely on the words of reputable Indigenous writers who have chosen to speak publicly from the cultural context to which they belong. Please note that parts of the book raise the matter of residential schools and other topics that may be distressing. I believe that there is value in trying to understand how people in Canada encounter and imagine sleep, and approaching such a topic requires attention to diverse experiences, including those that are positive as well as those that are painful.

This book was written primarily during my sabbatical in Vancouver on the unceded territory of the Coast Salish Peoples, including the territories of the xʷməθkwəy̓əm (Musqueam), Skwxwú7mesh (Squamish), and Səl'ílwətaʔ/Selilwitulh (Tsleil-Waututh) Nations. My writing has also taken place in Calgary on the traditional territories of the people of the Treaty 7 region and the home of the Métis Nation of Alberta, Region III, with additional ties to Athabasca University, located on Treaty 6 territory, the traditional territory of the Plains Cree, Woodland Cree, Beaver Cree, Saulteaux, Niisitapi (Blackfoot), Métis, and Nakota Sioux Peoples.

Portions of this book have appeared in other publications. The readings of *Slow War* and *The Marrow Thieves*, along with some commentary on critical sleep studies, appeared in "Stealing Sleep: Expanding the Conversation on the Literary Politics of Sleep and Insomnia," *English Studies in Canada* 44, no. 3 (2018): 67–89, for which I thank the anonymous referees and the journal's editorial team. Material adapted for chapter 1, along with a discussion transcript, appeared in "Sleep Through This Article: On Imagining Sleep in Canada," *Mosaic: An Interdisciplinary Critical Journal* 55, no. 1 (2022): 19–34; my thanks to Shepherd Steiner and the *Mosaic* team for arranging these conference proceedings. I am especially grateful to the two anonymous scholars who reviewed the full book manuscript with such generosity and expertise; their insights and encouragements were tremendously helpful. The book was written without assistance from generative AI, which came to prominence during my final revision stages. If this turns out to be one of the last books written without AI, I hope you enjoy its human flaws.

I also thank my kids, Holly and Jamie, for their lovely wit, for their willingness to appear in the book, and for teaching me so much about the benefits of sleeplessness. Finally, I thank you, my reader, for picking up this book, even if you quickly put it down again while you drift into slumber.

RESTLESS IN SLEEP COUNTRY

INTRODUCTION

Reading Sleep in a Restless World

HOW DID YOU SLEEP LAST NIGHT?

Unfortunately, if the many surveys and reports on this topic are any indication, the chances are worryingly high that your sleep was not great. For instance, nearly half of the participants in one sleep survey in Canada said that "they woke up feeling tired instead of refreshed."[1] When I read about this result, I thought, "My gosh! There are people who wake up feeling refreshed?" Sadly, I seem to have learned to see troubled sleep as an inevitability, and I'm certainly not the only one.

Public discourse around sleep tends to focus on the amount that we get each night, the upshot usually being that too many of us are sorely lacking in Zs, but whether you count yourself among the well-rested or the restless, there is more to sleep than quantity or even quality. Sleep is the source not only of replenishment and dreams but also of puzzling contradictions that carry a surprising amount of cultural weight.

One of the paradoxes of sleep is that this seemingly relaxed private activity is remarkably fraught with questions of cultural politics and power. A closely related paradox is that even though sleep is one of the most universal of all behaviours, it is tremendously revealing about the concerns of particular times and places. Yet another paradox is that even though sleep almost entirely evades direct experience, it is the subject of an incredible variety of deeply personal reflections and potent narratives, each of which develops its own perspective on the role of sleep in our lives.

Rather than asking the usual question "How did you sleep last night?" we might instead probe the cultural implications of sleep by asking, "What values were reflected in your sleep last night? For whom did you sleep? What did your sleep mean?" Even the question "Why do you sleep?" may involve more complexity than what is apparent at first glance. Moreover, we can move beyond a focus on individual slumbers by considering how sleep functions collectively as a contentious imaginative figure. Cultural visions of sleep are not merely incidental to the role that sleep plays in society but are intertwined with, and indeed shape, how we imagine and encounter sleep every day. A key message of this book is that we must learn to read such visions of sleep with care. We must develop a critical literacy of sleep in a restless world.

Defining sleep is surprisingly difficult, much like defining "life" or "time." Sleep is a form of suspended consciousness, but not all forms of suspended consciousness are sleep, and not all consciousness is suspended during sleep. Scientists define sleep in much the same way that they define death, through measurements of brainwaves, but whereas a dead person is highly unlikely to contradict the flat line on an EEG, a sleeper whose brain is being monitored will often disagree with the scientists about when, whether, or how they were sleeping during the scan.[2] In her study of the cultural history of EEGs, Sandra Huber notes that sleep and waking are not necessarily fully distinct from one another, observing that sleep may come and go within different parts of the brain at different times.[3] Sleep may be a universal experience, but whether we study it through electronic equipment or personal reflection, its nature remains largely mysterious. Saint Augustine famously said that he knew exactly what time was until the moment someone asked him to explain it.[4] If someone had ever asked him what sleep was, he would have had the same crisis all over again.

Even if we have a hard time saying exactly what sleep might be, contemporary life in the acceleration society goes hand in hand with a belief that sleep is in crisis, a problem that has been linked to various elements of modernity – electric lights, electronic screens, and 24/7 connectivity – with roots reaching back to the dawn of industrialization and clock-driven work shifts.[5] The Oxford introductory volume on sleep doesn't beat around the bush, declaring that "our treatment of sleep today is brutish ... It seems likely that we sleep less now than at any other time in our recent history."[6] Statistics Canada has also sounded the alarm, reporting that "short sleep duration and poor sleep quality are prevalent among Canadian adults."[7] A recent headline from the *Globe and Mail*, "Canadians Are Not Getting Enough Sleep – And That's a Big Problem," is enough to keep readers up at night.[8]

However, some scholars contest the notion that the trouble with sleep is peculiar to modernity or industrialization, even arguing that the conditions of sleep for many people today are better than ever.[9] Most researchers do tend to believe that there really is a modern sleep crisis brought about by a dangerous decline in sleep in recent decades, but sleep habits are quite difficult to measure, which has led to disagreements about whether the sleep crisis truly reflects a widespread deficiency of sleep or whether it is at least partly a kind of moral panic within societies that actually tend to sleep decently well on average. Another important complexity is that, although industrialized sleep in general may indeed be in crisis, the sleep of those who are impoverished may be especially at risk, as some evidence shows that "sleep duration and quality are even lower in developing countries and among the poor in rich countries."[10]

Moreover, there has never been a perfect or "natural" form of human sleep to which we might try to return. The work of historian A. Roger Ekirch, who found that people in preindustrial societies slept in two phases at night, with a period of wakefulness in between, has led some people to believe that segmented sleep is the "true" form of healthy human sleep and that electric lights (which brought about later bedtimes, leaving room for only a single period of sleep) have expelled us from the Eden of ideal slumber. However, other studies have found that Ekirch's observations reflect only certain societies at certain historical moments, that we don't know enough about the quality of sleep in past societies to make useful comparisons, and that there is likely no universal ideal form of sleep.[11] Literary scholar Benjamin Reiss notes that "because sleep is always governed by society's rules and environmental pressures as well as by physiological needs … the search for one unchanging 'natural' way to sleep seems unlikely to solve our current collective sleep frustrations."[12] Indeed, before you sigh too longingly for the golden slumbers of early modern Europeans, take a moment to think about the bedbugs, fleas, and lice.[13] Perhaps every unhappy sleep, so to speak, is unhappy in its own way.

What remains certain is that decent sleep, whatever form it might take, is vital for human well-being and that sleep (or a lack thereof) is an enormous everyday quandary and preoccupation. Perhaps you have seen the list of health problems said to be caused by not getting enough sleep? It reads almost like a list of *all* health problems: artery blockage, heart failure, cancer, stroke, obesity, infection, diabetes, infertility, injury, emotional volatility, dementia, depression, anxiety, suicidality, genetic damage – I could go on.[14] If you stay awake all night smoking cigarettes, maybe it's the staying awake that will kill you. Matthew Walker, the director of UC Berkeley's Center for Human Sleep Science, writes that "no facet of the human body is spared the crippling, noxious harm of sleep loss."[15] His book on the subject contains helpful chapter titles such as "Chapter 8: Cancer, Heart Attacks, and a Shorter Life."[16] Researchers don't always agree on the extent to which sleep loss is truly to blame for this extraordinary list of afflictions (and Walker himself has drawn some controversy), but the overall picture is indeed alarming.

Similarly, news stories and self-help articles that present sleep science to the public tend to foster a sense of anxiety and guilt about our lack of sleep hygiene. These stories cover many different angles, but the one thing that they tend to agree on is that, when it comes to sleep, you're doing it wrong. You work late? You don't clear your mind of stressful thoughts before bed? You haven't bought the latest sleep gadget? You should know better! You've been wearing blue-light-blocking glasses because they're the latest sleep gadget? They don't work; you're a fool. You haven't been taking power naps? You're failing to unlock your full potential. You do take naps? That could be Alzheimer's. Sleeping on your back while pregnant? You might kill your baby. Worrying about insomnia? That's a sure-fire cause of insomnia.[17] And the list of health repercussions keeps growing. A headline in *Forbes* reads, "Sleep Deprivation: Here's How Lack of Snooze Can Affect Your Walking, Balance."[18] Another headline warns, "Mothers Who Don't Get Enough Sleep Age More Rapidly, Study Finds," again joining the long, depressing tradition of experts who shame mothers over the demands of parenting.[19] As is the case with many predicaments under neoliberalism, we are presented with the idea that sleep loss is an individual problem, for which every unique person deserves particular blame. Never mind (we are told) the cultural forces that delimit personal agency; we are supposed to learn about the individual health dangers of sleep loss, and we must personally alter our lives in complex, neurotic ways to avoid them. No wonder sleep is a source of anxiety and stress for so many people.

Tied up in these omens and scoldings are deeply embedded values around gender, profit, and individualistic responsibility. In response to the crisis of sleep, a "sleep-industrial complex" offers consumers solutions ranging from pillows and apps to trendy espresso drinks.[20] A research group led by sociologist Sara Arber also notes that the frequent portrayal of sleep as a medical problem (rather than as a matter of culture) leads to more dependence on pharmaceuticals, which in turn have a close relationship to the requirement of capitalism that workers remain alert and productive.[21] Sleep products can be genuinely helpful in some cases, but they tend to conceal the ways that sleep deficiency is tied to structural issues and social inequities. A weighted blanket can do only so much when we are kept awake by persistent overwork, deficient social safety nets, and technologies designed to be addicting. Modern life tends to be highly stimulating, and the situation is similar to how people are presented with endless, convenient processed foods and then made to feel guilty that they don't eat well. Or, as feminist philosopher and political science scholar Cressida Heyes puts it, using another comparison, "sleep has taken over from sex in the popular imagination as a topic for cultural anxiety and thwarted need."[22] The world incessantly forces psychologically powerful images of sleep habits into our eyes and ears, implying that we are failing to measure up.

Nevertheless, despite the anxiety and guilt, sleep remains a source of profound pleasure and recuperation. Sleep comes to our attention not only through science, technology, and consumerism but also through our intimate encounters with sleep as a fundamental necessity of human life and as a profound bodily experience. In a recent global time-use survey, people rated sleep as one of the most enjoyable ways to spend time, ahead of hobbies, video games, playing sports, reading, listening to music, going to parties, and visiting friends.[23] Somewhat facetiously, we might find it remarkable that the average person prefers unconsciousness over just about any activity imaginable. (Does this finding say something profound about the value of sleep, something concerning about chronic sleep loss, or something terrifying about our failure to take pleasure in life?) More assuredly, the factors that link sleep with both extreme pleasure and extreme anxiety hint at the massively contested personal and cultural ground occupied by our seemingly indifferent naps and snoozes.

As some of these difficulties suggest, sleep is not as passive and unconcerned an activity as it might appear. The fact that sleep is a universal human need can foster the all-too-easy belief that sleep practices are merely biological or otherwise apolitical, but even if the latest sleep-tracking gadget might imply that our nightly slumber is purely a matter of individual choice and personal responsibility, sleep is a site of politics, culture, and power. As cultural theorist Jonathan Crary observes, "Sleep of course has a dense history, as does anything presumed to be natural."[24] Recognizing that we are caught up in this unfolding history is a key step in unravelling the cultural politics of sleep and in understanding sleep as both a personal experience and a product of imagination that requires forms of engagement beyond what can be provided by sleep-tracking apps, luxury mattresses, and brain scans, as valuable as these things may be in their own ways. Even if there never was an ideal society of perfect sleepers in the past, we nevertheless can and should investigate the troubles with slumber in our own time, not only with the goal of sleeping better but also to illuminate and confront the figure of sleep as a crucial site of struggle and gratification in our lives.

Sleep, then, presents a vital opportunity for intervention from the humanities, the home of critical literacy. Because sleep is culturally conditioned, the ways that it is represented in cultural narratives and imaginative texts of all kinds play a major role in shaping how we experience it, and the study of such representations can illuminate the politics and aesthetics of sleep across many contexts. As literary scholar Michael Greaney asserts in his book *Sleep and the Novel*, "One way in which we invent sleep ... is by writing about it."[25] Or, approaching from the other direction, scholar and poet Anne Carson observes that there are "different ways of reading sleep, different kinds of readers of sleep."[26] Reading works of literature and other texts about sleep is important both because thoughtful literary representations shape our visions of sleep in consequential ways and because understanding the cultural power of sleep requires us to exercise the literary methods of close reading and critical analysis. A sleep-tracking mattress might tell you that you missed out on a cycle of REM sleep during the night, but thoughtful readings of cultural visions of sleep can tell us what sleep means, or ought to mean, within the systems of value, power, and care that shape our lives. This book aims to show how the critical initiative brought about by such readings can build a larger cultural literacy of sleep.

The particular focus of this book has to do with cultures of sleep in Canada, partly because this is where my expertise lies and also because little work has previously been done to understand how sleep operates as an intricate, diverse, and contested figure within this nation. Specifically, I argue that representations of sleep in Canadian texts and Indigenous texts can in different ways profoundly challenge, reconstruct, affirm, and otherwise bring to critical awareness the cultural functioning of sleep and its associated configurations of power and thought. Meanwhile, the skills of critical discernment that emerge through this work will be useful not only in Canada but also in all places where sleep and culture interact. We might say that every narrative that touches on sleep can be understood as a sleep socialization story; every news article, phone app, or poem that engages with slumber tries, for better or worse, to indoctrinate us into a particular vision of sleep.[27] Lying down and closing our eyes is an act that carries surprisingly high stakes, and we must learn to read sleep with thoughtful attention and care.

CRITICAL SLEEP STUDIES AND THIS BOOK

An emerging field known as critical sleep studies allows us to examine the intricate and contested roles that sleep plays within cultural experiences, forms of representation, and social practices of all kinds. This field challenges us to re-examine the often silent assumptions about how we sleep, how we conceive of sleep, and how we might confront the cultural forces through which our inequitable encounters with sleep take shape. Such an approach holds great promise for illuminating the politics and aesthetics of sleep in Canada, especially since there has never been a sustained study of cultural and literary representations of sleep in this nation. As I explain in the next chapter, sleeping in Canada is both the same and not the same as sleeping somewhere else, and textual representations of all kinds can illuminate what is at stake in this country, and beyond, when sleep arises as a matter of concern in both its literal and figurative forms.

Previous studies of sleep in a variety of contexts have provided important insights that will be useful to keep in mind. Although the general need for lengthy, high-quality sleep cannot be denied, critical sleep scholars often take pride in dispelling the myth that an ideal form of human sleep exists.[28] As

Greaney observes, "sleep is a non-negotiable biological inevitability, but the parameters of sleep – when? where? with whom? for how long? – are all open to negotiation."[29] In his historical study of sleep norms, Reiss traces the set of cultural expectations that have come to govern sleep in modern Western societies. He finds, for instance, that the expectation of sleeping alone or only with a spouse not only on a schedule with little variation from season to season but also in a room that is dedicated for that purpose is a relatively recent cultural construct tied to "the invention of normal sleep in the nineteenth century," a period of time when industrialization reshaped sleep and time use around factory workers' shifts.[30] Reiss also identifies sleep as a site of domination since sleep deprivation has often been a key element of oppression in slavery.[31] The theft of sleep as a form of torture emphasizes the relationship between sleep and power, even while it underscores the fact that sleep is, without question, a biological necessity.

Sara Arber, a pre-eminent scholar in the sociology of sleep, has also found that sleep and sleep disorders are inextricably linked to societal structures and cultural norms, that "*where, why,* and *how* we sleep are all sociocultural matters ... all historically and culturally contingent."[32] Arber's research group has learned that sleep patterns are tied inequitably to gender, power, age, income, and social roles of various kinds.[33] The social expectation, for instance, that women should perform intensive daily caregiving (and should bear the emotional labour that goes with it) disproportionately harms their sleep by creating "an invisible 'workplace' at night," resulting in health inequities that cannot be solved by general public advice about the importance of maintaining good personal "sleep 'hygiene.'"[34]

Cultural theorist Jonathan Crary, in his influential book *24/7: Late Capitalism and the Ends of Sleep,* expands on the connection between sleep loss and cultural norms by arguing that sleep, as one of the last remaining modes of experience where our attention does not contribute to profitable activity, "subsists as one of the great human affronts to the voraciousness of contemporary capitalism."[35] He sees capitalism, as well as related processes like military expansion, as forces that seek to achieve the ultimate extermination of sleep altogether. Crary's argument is important, giving us the ability to consider how new technologies may further erode sleep's ability to provide a refuge from monetized digital services.[36] Nevertheless, we might maintain some skepticism about Crary's claims, not only about whether the extermination of sleep is possible but also about the degree to which portraying capitalism as an all-out assault on sleep risks glossing over the kinds of inequities identified by Arber's research group.

One challenge to the idea that the 24/7 society places us on a nonstop path toward the destruction of sleep comes from the Slow movement, which encourages people to intentionally reduce the perceived pace of life. Books such as Maggie Berg and Barbara K. Seeber's *The Slow Professor*, if often not explicitly about sleep, may support better restfulness by encouraging readers to move away from the frenzy of obsessive productivity. The Slow movement has great value, and we would do well to heed its advice in certain areas, but it tends to have a difficult time accounting for inequities. If tenured professors improve their sleep by taking Berg and Seeber's advice to "do less,"[37] their less privileged colleagues and students may be the ones to pay the price with late, stressful nights as they finish the latest draft of the curriculum assessment on their own and as they wait for the slow professors to respond to their emails, submit their reference letters, and finish that overdue peer review report. As I discuss in chapter 4, theorists of social acceleration such as Hartmut Rosa have identified further limitations to the kinds of initiatives promoted within the Slow movement.

A vision of restfulness closely related to the Slow movement comes from American artist and community organizer Tricia Hersey, the founder of the Nap Ministry, an organization that promotes rest as a form of resistance to grind culture. Whereas the Slow movement has an unfortunate history of glossing over inequities, Hersey's book *Rest Is Resistance* holds the politics of race at its centre. Arguing that "sleep deprivation is a racial and social justice issue," Hersey notes that although the exhausting demands of overwork may be socially pervasive, they are not socially equal – that "capitalism and white supremacy ... have used bodies as a tool for production, evil, and destruction for centuries."[38] Hersey asks her readers to rest – simply rest – not out of a desire to gain energy and be more productive but so as to embrace their humanity and refuse the racist foundations of exhaustion. "Rest is radical," she says, "because it disrupts the lie that we are not doing enough."[39] One of the key difficulties with the Slow movement, namely that the very people who are oppressed by poverty and racism will likely be among the most severely punished for slowing down and doing less, is a central point of both worry and affirmation for Hersey. "The desperate and valid question of 'How can I rest, if I have to pay bills?'" she says, "is the beating heart of this work ... Resting as a form of resistance will be part of a lifelong unraveling."[40] Hersey's book embodies a key point in critical sleep studies: despite being universal, sleep is profoundly tied to the politics of equity and justice.

In his book *The Politics of Sleep*, British sociologist Simon J. Williams provides a useful foundation for what might be called the central tenets of critical sleep studies, making the key argument that because sleep is inevitably tied to power relations, controversy, regulation, and critique, sleep "is political through and through."[41] For Williams, current discourse about sleep can be categorized as belonging either to the "sleep-negative agenda," where sleep is neglected, invalidated, privatized, and depoliticized, to the "sleep-positive agenda," where sleep and sleep loss are recognized as important matters of social concern, or to the "critical-reflexive agendas," which investigate how sleep is governed, politicized, and tied to injustices.[42] Williams notes that these agendas are shifting and complex; he observes, for example, that even if the sleep-positive agenda brings about genuine efforts to protect sleep, it also tends to foster a perhaps too-cozy relationship between public health warnings about sleep loss and the growing consumer sleep industry. And although we might be tempted to see the humanities and social sciences as ready participants in the critical-reflexive and sleep-positive agendas, Williams argues that the traditional neglect of sleep within these disciplines also makes them complicit in the sleep-negative agenda.[43] Indeed, as *The Slow Professor* and *Rest Is Resistance* indicate, the neglect of sleep at universities goes beyond the lack of attention to sleep as a subject matter; Hersey asserts that academia, with its long hours and urgent deadlines, "is the headquarters for grind culture."[44]

Williams's classification of agendas gives us a powerful rubric for assessing sleep discourse, and various scholars have taken up his terminology in productive ways. For example, in their study of sleep-tracking apps and gadgets, cultural theorist Diletta De Cristofaro and philosopher Simona Chiodo argue that the Oura sleep-tracking ring, which presents users with detailed data on their sleep stages and heart rate, may not be as "sleep-positive" a tool as it appears. "Ultimately," they assert, the ring "upholds an instrumental view of rest as a tool for maximising productivity, performance, and achievement during the day."[45] In this sense, products that appear to promote good sleep may actually perpetuate a sleep-negative agenda, even contributing to "a crisis of subjectivity" as users' understanding of their own identity becomes tied up in the charts and graphs of the "Quantified Self."[46] Like De Cristofaro and Chiodo, I draw from, and sometimes complicate, Williams's rubric throughout this book. His assertion that sleep "is political through and through" doesn't require us to concede that sleep has no existence beyond politics – sleep, after all, was biologically essential long before the evolution of humans and our concerns – but if we want to think carefully about the function of sleep in our lives, we need to foster a deep political awareness.

When it comes to material objects, the politics of sleep can be illuminated not only through studies of high-tech sleep-tracking gadgets but also by examining commonplace items such as blankets and beds. Literary scholar Hilary Hinds, for instance, has shown that the choice of a bed is not merely a matter of comfort and price but additionally reflects shifting cultural visions of family relationships and other values. She focuses on the history of the twin bed, showing how the rise of twin beds for married couples in Britain starting in the late nineteenth century and their fall from grace in the second half of the twentieth century reflected and shaped changing notions of "hygiene, modernity and marriage."[47] Sleep objects that I discuss in later chapters include mattresses, pillows, and phones resting on nightstands.

Indigenous scholars reflect a diversity of perspectives on sleep, often emphasizing the importance of dreams. Such work includes Leanne Betasamosake Simpson's study of Anishinaabe ways of learning through dreaming, as well as Willie Ermine's study of dreams as a central element of Indigenous epistemology. Ermine, a scholar from the Sturgeon Lake First Nation in Saskatchewan, notes that the spirit, which is a key point of access for knowledge, "is the haven of dreams, those peculiar images that flash symbolic messages to the knower."[48] In Canada, the cultural significance of these perspectives persists in its own right, even though Indigenous experiences of sleep have become entwined with the politics of colonization due to the settler society's frequent efforts to extinguish traditional Indigenous sleeping arrangements. I discuss these concerns in more detail in later chapters.

Scholars in literary studies have examined representations of the act of sleep as well as the function of sleep as a culturally contested figure. Lee Scrivner offers a brief survey of sleep in the Western literary canon, from Greek myth to Shakespeare and beyond. He notes that sleep has often been represented as a void or a mere absence of agency, a characterization that fell out of favour after EEG technology offered a glimpse into the startling amount of activity in the sleeping brain.[49] He also traces how the ability to induce sleep has been associated with magic and power, as in the case of the poisoned apple in *Snow White*.[50] Garrett Sullivan focuses more specifically on the representation of sleep and vitality in early modern texts like Shakespeare's *Henry IV* and *Henry V*, Milton's *Paradise Lost*, and Dryden's *All for Love*. He argues that these texts use sleep as a vehicle for "exploring different models of humanness," all borrowing from the Aristotelian notion of the tripartite soul.[51]

In his more contemporary study, Reiss suggests that "since sleep is such an intimate, even hidden, aspect of human experience, it requires a literary focus on interior states to draw out its history."[52] He argues that the literary focus on the intimacies of sleep can expand outward to develop critical questions about cultures of sleep as a whole. Works of fiction, film, and other imaginative texts are particularly useful in that "they present contemporary sleep troubles not as a personal problem to be managed by pills and experts, but as a social, economic, and environmental one."[53] However, in studying art, literature, and news media reports, Heyes has found that "representations of sleep are increasingly deployed within existing scripts of class, race, and gender stratification."[54] Emerging from these two different assertions – that narratives of sleep can either question or reinforce cultural assumptions – is the need for us to develop skills of discernment in figuring out which narratives do what kinds of representational work.

In his book *Sleep and the Novel*, Greaney examines the cultural construction of sleep as perceived in works of fiction ranging from Jane Austen's *Sense and Sensibility* to twenty-first-century stories that cast a skeptical eye on sleep laboratories. Beginning with the central assertion that "one way in which we invent sleep ... is by writing about it," Greaney comes to see the novel as "a notable record of the diverse and contradictory *valuations* of sleep in relation to wakefulness that have circulated in modern culture."[55] Novels variously render sleep invisible, treat it as an act of negligence, or position it "as an ideal standard by which the futile busyness of waking life might be judged."[56]

These scholars provide groundbreaking insights that show how sleep must be understood in terms of narrative representation, yet their work also leaves much territory to be explored. Existing literary studies, for example, often focus on white authors, who are usually male, raising unanswered questions about the visions of sleep that emerge from a greater diversity of writers, as well as about how literary representations of sleep might intervene in matters of gender, race, colonization, and other concerns. Indeed, these studies might inspire us to ask a variety of further questions: What *else* is happening in novels that involve sleep? What more can we learn from other literary forms such as poetry? And how might we build a larger cultural literacy of sleep by using the skills of literary studies to examine other kinds of texts and practices, from movies and advertisements to the use of luxury mattresses?

This is not a comprehensive survey, but it introduces some of the key concepts that I wish to apply. The fields of critical sleep studies and literary studies have only just begun to cross paths, and developing the interactions between these approaches promises to bring about startling insights. Sleep – as a figure, an act, a metaphor, a bodily ache, a desire, a frustration, a form of currency and power – operates as a profound and often invisible force within our cultural worlds and individual lives, yet only a few studies have examined how, why, and to what ends sleep functions in diverse texts. The representation of sleep in Canadian and Indigenous works in particular has not been engaged in any sustained way, meaning that sleep has tended to operate invisibly, behind closed doors, as it were. By peeking beneath the covers, I hope to deepen the existing critical approaches to sleep in literature in order to show that we have much to gain by applying the methods of critical sleep studies to diverse contemporary texts. After all, the notion that sleep is "culturally contingent" raises many questions about how such contingencies operate, not just in sociological terms but also within the realm of figurative representation. Focusing on sleep in Canadian and Indigenous texts can help to counter the so-called sleep-negative agenda by developing a consciousness of sleep as a vital and contested site of representation, thereby opening up a variety of possibilities for critical-reflexive interventions and allowing us to test the uneasy ground of sleep-positive perspectives. Thoughtful readings of diverse texts can inspire us to move beyond superficial notions of whether a given work is "for" or "against" good sleep by embracing a more nuanced sense of critical discernment.

Many of the literary works that I discuss – such as Cherie Dimaline's *The Marrow Thieves* (a dystopian novel by a female Métis writer about surviving colonization) and Benjamin Hertwig's *Slow War* (a work of contemporary war poetry by a white, male veteran of the Afghanistan War) – can be read as critical-reflexive works in the sense that they insist that sleep be seen as both a vital act and a cultural site that is under attack by systemic forces. When read in this way, such texts can also be said to complicate what it means for a text to be sleep-positive; if sleep is not a single natural thing but a complex cluster of acts, concepts, and figures, then more nuanced positions are required than the simple advocation of good sleep. These texts attempt to sort out contested cultural visions of sleep, seeking to protect or resist such visions in accordance with complex matters of justice and power. Other texts and practices that I discuss, such as Sleep Country Canada ads and bedtime phone apps, test our ability to read sleep by presenting visions of slumber that are internally conflicted yet have massive cultural and economic reach. Approaching such works thoughtfully can sharpen our awareness of how visions of sleep shape our everyday world, intertwining with matters of systemic power, the commercialization of private moments, and the genuine pleasures to be found when we lay our heads on our pillows and let consciousness dissolve.

Thus, rather than simply categorizing texts within a rubric, close readings can add more subtlety to our understanding of what kinds of forces are in operation and how figurative representation can play a central role in identifying and responding to them. Greaney's assertion that we invent sleep by writing about it, like so many useful arguments, seems self-evident once it is laid out in front of us, and although his study tends to focus on sleep in terms of how it is valued or devalued in its relationship to wakefulness, the invention of sleep involves many other complexities, not least of which is the question of who constitutes the "we" who do the inventing. Many visions of sleep have been silenced on the cultural stage, and critical sleep studies, even more than many other fields, is in need of greater engagement from more diverse voices. I hope to play a role here in expanding the scope of the field by investigating how sleep circulates within the cultural landscape in Canada, taking into account practices and representations that emerge from many different positions of value and power.

This book begins with an examination of how sleep functions in Canada, moves on to a study of the power of literary narratives to shape how sleep is understood culturally, and then offers a larger vision of how narratives of all kinds can condition how we experience sleep amidst widespread concerns such as pandemic responses, technology, and the climate crisis. The first chapter, "Welcome to Sleep Country," examines cultures of sleep in Canada. Drawing from sleep surveys, historical studies, memoirs, and visual art, I offer an overview of the key issues that arise when we ask how people imagine and encounter sleep within this nation. By way of a case study, I examine recent advertisements from bedding supply retailer Sleep Country Canada. One key ad, titled "Sleep Is for the Strong," follows the sleep-deprived life of an exhausted office worker who buys a new mattress. Although this narrative may appear to place value on sleep, the ad in fact promotes sleep only for the purpose of maintaining the worker's exhausting schedule. This focus means that sleep, as a product, is both the antidote to and the enabler of the insomniac 24/7 society. The hazards lurking within such everyday representations can teach us how sleep circulates as a contested figure in Canada, a matter that requires us to build a critical literacy of sleep and to seek out other forms of narrative and representation that might allow us to imagine sleep differently.

Chapter 2, "The Poetics of Sleep," argues that if we want to become careful readers of sleep, literature is worth our time. Literature can teach us to see sleep with fresh eyes and with a keen awareness of how sleep, as a conceptual figure, can push and pull our attention in many directions. A difficulty with sleep is that, because it cannot necessarily be directly perceived, it is difficult to represent in narrative form. Poetry provides a key intervention in this problem, and this chapter examines representations of sleep in poetry in Canada. Poetry about sleep tests the limits of literary representation, and it speaks to the complex cultural role of sleep by developing aesthetic, philosophical, and political visions of sleep, by commenting on the need for literature itself to engage with sleep, and by building a larger picture of the contested ways that sleep has been imagined in this nation. After examining works by a. rawlings, Dionne Brand, Alootook Ipellie, and others, I end the chapter with a close reading of Hertwig's book *Slow War*. By challenging dominant representations of sleep in the context of war, *Slow War* reclaims sleep from the figurative realm and brings it back to the literal.

Whereas poetry tends to experiment with elements of language and form, narrative fiction more often explores thematic concerns around sleep, frequently to do with inequity and trauma but also involving healing, intimacy, and growth. Chapter 3, "Fictions of Sleep," examines representations of sleep in fiction from Canada, showing how the dreams and slumbers in these narratives negotiate a particular set of social values, expectations, and histories. I open the chapter with a reading of disrupted sleep in Joshua Whitehead's novel *Jonny Appleseed* in the context of Two-Spirit identity, intolerance, and poverty. I then consider the links between sleep, gender, and race through readings of works such as the novels *Brother* by David Chariandy and *The English Patient* by Michael Ondaatje, and I examine how the representation of narcolepsy in Nino Ricci's novel *Sleep* develops the link between sleep and identity. To examine more diverse narrative forms, I consider the apocalyptic film *Awake*, in which a global disaster takes away people's ability to sleep, and Suzanne Buffam's genre-defying work *A Pillow Book*, which invites an investigation of the cultural role of the pillow. I end this chapter with a close reading of Cherie Dimaline's postapocalyptic novel *The Marrow Thieves*, in which the settler society attempts to steal the sleep and dreams of the Indigenous characters. Literary visions of sleep thus identify the aesthetic possibilities of the literary imagination, and they also illuminate the nature of the cultural world – with all its possibilities and hazards – from which such an imagination might spring.

A brief interlude titled "Sleeping through Covid-19" shows how the Covid-19 pandemic, especially the sudden lockdowns that occurred throughout most of the world in early 2020, can illuminate some of the key issues at stake in how sleep operates as both practice and representation, as both a bodily need tied to social concerns and a form of manipulation and power. After considering how the pandemic and the lockdowns impacted literal sleep in highly inequitable ways, I examine figurative representations of sleep during the lockdowns, focusing especially on an advertisement from Mazda Canada called "Sleeping Roads." This ad reveals how the figure of sleep can play a key role in the crucial debate over whether society could or should return to "normal" after the pandemic. Reading sleep in this kind of ad can foster the critical skills necessary for responding to the ideological visions embedded within images of slumber across texts and media of all kinds.

Whereas chapters 2 and 3 focus on the ability of literary narratives to shape cultural visions of sleep, with the interlude offering an example of how representations of sleep can intervene in crucial public debates, the final two chapters extend the importance of narrative and representation to the pervasive concerns of technology and the climate crisis. Chapter 4, "Entering

Sleep Mode," asks what it means to live with technologies of sleep, particularly as embodied by the utopian idea that any sleep problem must have a technological solution – that the same technologies that helped to create the problem will now solve it. What is needed, I argue, is not a rejection of technology or scientific curiosity but a critical literacy of sleep objects (and the discourse surrounding them) that accounts for our messy encounters with complex products, interventions, and representations. I further argue that if we want to understand the products that shape our sleep, we need to engage closely with matters of narrative. In particular, I consider the phenomenon of Sleep Stories, bedtime stories for adults produced by Calm, a relaxation-focused phone app. Canadian writer Chris Advansun, although unknown to most scholars, is a Sleep Story writer whose works have been downloaded millions of times by sleepy phone users. I consider the function, form, and cultural politics of Sleep Stories, both through critical analysis and through an account of my own attempt to fall asleep to them. I end the chapter with a close reading of Sandra Huber's poetry, which takes the shape of an EEG graph, providing surprising glimpses into what it might mean for us to perceive sleep in its own right.

Chapter 5, "Sleeping in the Anthropocene," examines the implications of ecological crisis for sleep in a warming and inequitable world. I start with an account of my family's experience during the Calgary flood of 2013, which resulted in sleepless nights for us and many others, and I consider the larger health costs of global heating in terms of sleep. I then turn to climate fiction, arguing that if we want to learn how to approach sleep in the age of climate collapse, we need to see how different forms of imaginative representation can reshape our thinking. I conclude the chapter with three examples of how such ecological readings of sleep can take shape, emerging from three very different forms: poetry by Rita Wong, temporary "landwork" photography by Marlene Creates, and comics by Simon Orpana. In their diversity, these works show how the business of thinking through sleep in the Anthropocene cannot be reduced to a singular vision or framework. In their specificity, each text proposes its own model for developing a literacy of sleep in a world of ecological and cultural complexity, hazards, and beauty.

The book's brief conclusion, "The Work of Sleep," returns to the practical question of how we might sleep better. Self-help books will tell you to avoid caffeine and to lower your room temperature, but individual behaviour can go only so far in addressing structural problems; fostering better sleep for everyone depends on cultural changes. Critical sleep studies gives us the tools to engage in such interventions, and the skills that emerge from literary analysis and cultural studies allow us to see sleep through fresh eyes, both within Canada and beyond. Indeed, the cultural and literary politics of sleep will extend far beyond the texts and practices discussed in this book, and more voices are needed in order to deepen our critical visions of sleep. To help spark your own investigations of sleep, I provide an appendix with sample exercises for reimagining sleep in a restless world. In this way, I hope to encourage you to keep learning how to read the sleep socialization stories that you encounter each day.

My project thus has three central goals: to illuminate the cultural figure of sleep in Canada, in all its inequities, pleasures, and hope; to offer a guidebook that can help us all to develop a critical literacy of sleep informed by an awareness of cultural politics and the nuances of many forms of representation; and to offer an invitation for a greater diversity of readers to further deepen the field. Sleep may be a universal act, but it is shaped in surprising ways by different experiences, even while it shapes many elements of our world in turn, and these factors deserve to be understood from a multitude of perspectives. Whether you have already fallen asleep while reading this introduction or whether you stay awake until the end, my hope is that this book will inspire you to decide what kind of reader of sleep you might wish to become.

1

Welcome to Sleep Country

CULTURES OF SLEEP IN CANADA

SLEEPING IN CANADA is both the same and not the same as sleeping somewhere else. There is nothing unique about the physical act of sleep in Canada: the intense bodily need for good-quality slumber and the stages of REM and non-REM sleep that revolve in a cycle throughout the night are universal elements of sleep. Yet, because sleep is never a purely natural act but is expressed through cultural forms of meaning and value, sleeping in Canada is shaped within particular social expectations and histories that occur nowhere else.

A large percentage of adults in Canada, perhaps as much as half the population, report some degree of trouble sleeping, with insomnia symptoms being most prevalent in women, in people with lower levels of education and income, and in people who report having poor health or a poor quality of life.[1] Statistics Canada warns that "poor sleep quality and high sleep variability are common," noting that widespread efforts to improve sleep quality and duration are needed for meeting health objectives.[2] Moreover, the prevalence of insomnia in Canada is not stable over time but has apparently been increasing dramatically since at least 2002.[3] The problem of sleep loss for adolescents, meanwhile, may be even worse, with social media apps and early school hours taking much of the blame. The director of sleep medicine at Toronto's Hospital for Sick Children offers the gloomy prediction that "in 20 years time, we're going to see a whole generation of adults who are functioning sub-optimally."[4] As a result, the alarming news headlines keep piling up. "Canadians Are Not Getting Enough Sleep," says the *Globe and Mail*. "Lack of Sleep Is 'Epidemic' among Canadian Teens," declares CBC *News*.[5]

In emphasizing the most catastrophic data, it is easy to lose sight of the fact that most people actually sleep quite well. The same Statistics Canada report cited above notes that "three-quarters of Canadian adults meet the sleep duration recommendations."[6] And although teens may be pushed toward sleep deprivation due to social factors, young people tend to sleep well when given the chance, with insomnia symptoms being less prevalent in children and adolescents than in adults.[7] These glimmers of good news don't make up for the painful sleep loss that millions of people experience, but they can help to rein in the most calamitous interpretations of the sleep crisis.

Alongside a tendency to focus on the most alarming figures, another reason for the difficulty in assessing people's sleep is that self-reported sleep data are notoriously unreliable. Survey results provide a helpful glimpse into the bedrooms of the nation, but they also raise questions about how people's perceptions of their own sleep may reflect multiple factors. When Statistics Canada reports a striking 42 per cent increase in insomnia symptoms between 2007 and 2015, surely this finding reflects a real problem that requires attention, with the obvious suspects of smartphones, overwork, and stress perhaps taking much of the blame.[8] To what extent, however, have the waters been muddied by shifting definitions of insomnia, by the difficulties with measuring insomnia symptoms, and by the moral panic around living in a sleep-deprived society? Neurologist W. Chris Winter notes that many self-reported insomniacs appear to be excellent snoozers under objective measurement, but they "have made up their minds that they are bad sleepers."[9] This "insomnia identity" really does impair daytime functioning, and it is just one of many issues that cannot easily be perceived through surveys.[10]

Compounded with these factors is the tendency of time-use surveys to confusingly lump sleep together with other languid activities. Statistics Canada reports that Canadians aged sixty-five and over spend nine hours each day "sleeping, resting, relaxing," or "sick in bed,"[11] ambiguously conflating sleep with insomnia, boredom, and illness. And the thorny nuances don't stop there. The reporting on gender and income levels implies that sleep loss is often tied to, among other things, gaps in social safety nets; we should take this result seriously and act on it, but what do we make of the fact that a survey showing that women "were more likely to report trouble falling asleep or staying asleep" also shows that men sleep fewer hours than women on average?[12] This information may point to a gendered distinction between insomnia (the inability to sleep) and sleep deprivation (sleep loss imposed by external factors or self-imposed as a matter of choice). However, the distinction between insomnia and sleep deprivation is not necessarily clear-cut since external factors can lead to stress that causes insomnia. Meanwhile, experts don't necessarily agree on the amount of sleep that people of different demographics should get in the first place. Immense complexities are involved in untangling the unequal allocations and experiences of sleep across society.

Certain occupations also carry their own sleep hazards. People in medical professions, for instance, while engaged in caring for the health of others, often must neglect their own health due to demanding workloads and long hours. A Canadian study during the Covid-19 pandemic found that nurses, who endure chronic stress and frequent rotations between day and night shifts, tended to get less sleep than other people – and when they did sleep, their sleep tended to be lighter, with less time spent in vital REM stages.[13] Monitoring devices on the nurses' bodies showed that the cardiovascular stress response that impairs sleep and damages the heart persisted even after several days off at the end of a rotation. Studies in the United States (potentially with implications for Canada) have found that doctors, particularly males, "report hallucinations, life-threatening seizures, depression and suicide due to sleep deprivation."[14] Physicians and medical students must work exhausting hours under immense stress, sometimes enduring twenty-eight-hour shifts, leading some doctors to "kill themselves for fear of harming a patient as a result of their extreme sleep deprivation."[15] Even beyond the medical professions, people whose jobs involve providing round-the-clock services for others may be especially vulnerable, with high rates of sleep loss reported, for example, among taxi drivers and hotel housekeeping staff.[16] Nevertheless, occupational sleep hazards can extend across all ranks of privilege, especially in high-pressure workplaces; one group at risk of dangerous overuse of pharmaceutical sleep aids is National Hockey League players, who are sometimes pressured into taking what former Vancouver Canuck Tom Sestito calls an "insane" amount of Ambien in order to maintain top physical performance amidst exhausting travel schedules.[17]

Across the different regions of Canada, sleep statistics often appear fairly uniform at first glance. People in Quebec, for instance, seem to get a few minutes more sleep on average than those in Ontario, an interesting but subtle variation.[18] On closer examination, however, certain regional differences can be surprisingly pronounced and difficult to assess, raising more complex questions. A study in 2021 revealed that an alarming 24 per cent of seniors in New Brunswick "take sleeping pills on a regular basis – far above the national average of seven per cent."[19] The Atlantic provinces overall have a higher rate of sleeping pill use, whereas Saskatchewan has the lowest. Researchers are at a loss to explain the reasons for these disparities, other than declaring them a matter of culture and habituation, but the consequences may be profound. In addition to carrying a risk of dependence, sleeping pills can create problems with memory loss, poor balance, and impaired driving – problems for which seniors are already at heightened risk. Meanwhile, Statistics Canada typically does not distribute sleep surveys to First Nations reserves or to sparsely populated regions, leaving appreciable gaps in the overall data.[20] These gaps mean that whereas some populations in Canada show sleep troubles that are difficult to assess, other populations, often among the most marginalized, are excluded from the published assessments altogether.

As with the modern sleep crisis, discussed in the introduction, it is reasonable to conclude that sleep loss is indeed a serious problem in Canada, with a great many people suffering from sleep deprivation or a consistent inability to sleep. Sleep patterns are difficult to measure, and focusing only on the most alarming statistics would be misleading, but the pervasiveness and inequities of sleep loss are deeply troubling, especially given their repercussions for overall well-being. We do need to act on the inequities of sleeplessness, and we need to hold sleep loss to account for its contributions to long-term health problems, not to mention for the everyday ailments of tiredness and fatigue.

Surveys and statistics are vitally important for recognizing trends and pointing the way toward interventions. Such tools, however, can never tell the whole story, and we must turn to other sources to further grasp how troubles with sleep circulate within, and in some ways define, social experiences in Canada. Diverse personal narratives and historical accounts, for instance, can illuminate the cultural politics of sleep in vital ways, sometimes drawing attention to distressing links between sleep and power.

Indeed, the manipulation of sleep as a form of oppression is closely tied to some of the nation's worst injustices. In *Clearing the Plains*, a historical study of the Canadian government's brutal use of starvation and disease to control Indigenous Peoples on the Prairies, James Daschuk notes that "while reserve conditions were deplorable, the long-term ill health of the Indigenous population became increasingly defined by the growing Indian residential school system. For decades, overcrowding, poor nutrition, and neglect contributed to systemic TB infection among children who attended the institutions."[21] The link between overcrowded living quarters and tuberculosis within the schools was understood at the time, which means that inadequate sleeping arrangements served in effect as a genocidal tool for the Canadian suppression of Indigenous Peoples. One physician, registering alarm at the rampant illness in the schools, wrote in 1895 that "one of the first things to do towards lessening the amount of Tuberculosis is to relieve the over-crowded condition of the School. Additional sleeping and class room accommodation should be immediately provided."[22] Such pleas were ignored, along with the voices of Indigenous families themselves, for generations. The lack of awareness or concern among non-Indigenous Canadians about the genocidal actions of their own government toward Indigenous Peoples is a well-understood failure of the Canadian education system and public sphere, one that is only now being gradually and inconsistently addressed. That the colonizing society saw fit to force Indigenous children into sleeping quarters guaranteed to contribute to widespread deadly illness is one of many shameful parts of this history.

An incident in Thunder Bay, Ontario, in 2021 illuminates how the sleep of Indigenous people continues to be uniquely policed, also hinting at how sleep can serve as a flashpoint in the context of systemic racism. One evening in April, a city transit officer found two Indigenous men sleeping on a bench at the City Hall transit terminal.[23] Rather than talking with the men or leaving them alone, the officer pulled out his phone, took pictures of them, and then called over a few other transit drivers and a security guard who also started taking photos while pointing and laughing at the sleeping men. An Indigenous mother and her young son who witnessed the incident took to social media to share their dismay at this treatment of the sleeping men, with the wide circulation of the story resulting in public outrage, news media reports, and an investigation by the city. The power dynamic of city officers confronting Indigenous people within the context of systemic colonial racism was compounded here by the power that those who are awake and watching hold over those who are asleep and watched. However, the vulnerability of the men's sleep also became a vital factor in determining that the transit officers' actions would be met with public condemnation rather than indifference. If the two men had been awake, they still would have had little recourse in that moment in terms of their position as racialized subjects confronted by officers of the city, yet their position of powerlessness became heightened, and fully visible, by virtue of their sleep.

After the issue erupted on social media, the transit drivers' union argued that drivers are made to endure daily verbal and physical abuse, that they sometimes take photos to help with the issuing of trespassing notices, and that they often hesitate to approach people in distress due to the very fear of having their actions circulated without context on social media.[24] The union also called for more government funding for shelters and mental health supports. Transit drivers are surely in a difficult position, but in this case the apparent laughing and pointing quickly reduced the situation to a matter of racist conduct. In this regard, the public condemnation was a rightful response, yet a social media storm is unlikely to approach the larger issue with the care that it requires. Like so many confrontations, this event was not an isolated moment but occurred in the context of generations of oppressive colonial power. Sleep played a surprisingly central role here in that it facilitated both the racist act and the social-media-fuelled denunciation that followed. This incident gives us the chance to see sleep as a clarifying lens, both for colonial oppression and for the ambivalent nature of fleeting public outrage.

Colonization can also be understood to play a significant role in the climate crisis, which has its own implications for sleep. Indigenous philosopher and environmental justice professor Kyle Powys Whyte, a member of the Citizen Potawatomi Nation in Oklahoma, notes that the linked forces of colonialism and capitalism ushered in the "carbon-intensive economics" behind global heating.[25] Whyte argues that the vulnerability of Indigenous societies to climate change can thus be understood "as an intensification of colonially-induced environmental changes";[26] the actions of colonial societies in degrading ecosystems and forcing Indigenous Peoples to leave their ancestral lands can be said to foreshadow the damages and forced migrations associated with climate collapse. Among the many other repercussions of the climate crisis for Indigenous Peoples, rising temperatures affect sleep in various ways. In her memoir *The Right to Be Cold*, Inuit environmental advocate and political representative Sheila Watt-Cloutier describes how the shrinking ice and melting snows brought about by global heating are making traditional Inuit ways of life untenable. She quotes Lucas Ittulak of Nain, Newfoundland and Labrador, who observes that the snow "is no good for igloos anymore. [Twenty years ago] we used to be able to stop anywhere we needed a place to sleep just to build an igloo and sleep in that. And nowadays you can't just find good snow anywhere."[27] Watt-Cloutier points out that tents make a poor substitute for traditional Inuit snow houses during hunting trips; tents are bulky and burdensome, and they don't "provide adequate insulation in the winter cold or protection from bears."[28] The threat that the climate crisis poses to traditional Inuit sleeping arrangements during hunting trips is thus both a serious practical problem and a microcosm of the larger threats to Indigenous societies brought about by the colonial regime of fossil fuels.

Published memoirs from writers in Canada thus provide another way of moving beyond the impersonal charts and graphs of statistical analyses, offering windows into the lived experiences of sleep that emerge in a diverse and inequitable nation. We might trace this back at least as far as Catharine Parr Traill's account of her life as a settler in Ontario in the early nineteenth century, where her list of "the most useful articles for a settler to bring out" from England includes only four entries: tools, clothing, shoes, and "good bedding, especially warm blankets."[29] The memoirs of Traill's sister Susanna Moodie show a particular obsession with sleeplessness as an ailment for new settlers. She speaks of backwoodsmen who sleep perilously in front of open fireplaces, their "bedding often riddled with holes made by hot particles of wood flying out during the night."[30] Moodie herself is constantly kept awake by sounds and anxieties as she navigates the difficulties of pioneer life; her memoir includes an exasperated poem called "Oh, Let Me Sleep!"[31] When her house catches fire, her first thought is to save the bedding.[32]

Unscientifically, these accounts might prompt us to question the notion that those of us in the twenty-first century deserve special sympathy for the modern crisis of sleep in a technology-driven world, lending support instead to the idea that problems with sleep circulate in their own ways across different places and times. In addition to recording the harsh conditions of settler life, such narratives can show how expectations around sleep reveal cultural values tied to individualism, class status, and the infrastructure of everyday life. Moodie quotes her friend Tom, who complains that "there is no such thing as privacy in this country. In the bush, all things are in common; you cannot even get a bed without having to share it with a companion. A bed on the floor in a public sleeping-room! Think of that; a public sleeping-room! – men, women, and children, only divided by a paltry curtain. Oh, ye gods!"[33] Tom lays it on pretty thick, but those of us who are accustomed to private bedrooms can sympathize with his sleep troubles, and we can see how his English roots and class consciousness make for a difficult adjustment to settler life. Stepping back from his immediate experience, however, we might draw a disturbing comparison between the public sleeping-room and the conditions imposed in the overcrowded residential schools in later decades. Whereas Moodie and her publisher saw fit to circulate Tom's horrified reaction to the sleeping-room, the settler society at large would remain silent on the more abject sleeping conditions in the schools. In the collective consciousness, some people's sleep matters more than the sleep of others.

Moreover, the comments by Traill and Moodie about the "backwoods" of early Canada, like many such narratives, are examples of how settler accounts of the "New World" served to silence and distort Indigenous cultures and ways of life, even while settlers demonstrated incredible resourcefulness and perseverance in difficult conditions. Traill recounts a story about a settler widow who is shocked when an Indigenous man arrives at her house at night during a heavy snowfall. At first, she fears that he will murder her children, but when he turns out to act peacefully, she is so relieved that she offers him her own bed for the night. "It was evident," Traill writes, that "the Indian had never seen, and certainly never reposed on, an European bed. After a mute examination of the bed-clothes for some minutes, with a satisfied laugh, he sprang upon the bed, and, curling himself up like a dog, in a few minutes was sound asleep."[34] Such an account is deeply troubling not only for how it represents the man – his ignorance and incivility, his being compared to a dog, his astonishing failure to be murderous – but also for its lack of curiosity about the sleeping practices and ways of life that had by then already existed for thousands of years beyond the doors of the settler's log cabin. As I discuss later, Indigenous Peoples have often approached sleep and dreams with deep respect as sources of insight and cultural strength, a practice that is deftly erased in accounts such as Traill's.

In twenty-first-century memoirs, struggles with sleep continue to emerge in many forms, often tied to problematic cultural norms and incomplete social safety nets. Calgary writer Teresa Wong's graphic memoir *Dear Scarlet:*

The Story of My Postpartum Depression gives an illustrated account of her intense struggle with postpartum depression after the birth of her first child. As Wong battles overwhelming hopelessness and feelings of inadequacy, the extreme pain of her depression is compounded by the failures of the social environment that is supposed to support her as a new mother. Doctors, nurses, and friends tend to quickly dismiss her comments about being depressed, telling her that she will soon get over the "baby blues" and that she should "focus on the positive."[35] Continual sleep deprivation permeates and intensifies this experience, and when Wong (told to nap when the baby naps) is granted occasional short periods of rest, she lies awake running through a litany of anxious self-doubts, even to the point of thinking that her baby would be better off without her.

In one scene, the baby's incessant crying during the night leads Wong to say to her husband, "I think I hate her," to which her husband replies, "She's just a little baby." Wong then writes in a caption above her sleep-deprived self, "He was right. I didn't hate you. I hated myself."[36] This rapid spiral of dark thoughts emphasizes the way that sleep deprivation can so easily be linked to depression and the distortion of judgment, as Wong takes a mere three panels to undertake a harrowing sequence from hating her baby to hating herself. The simplicity and spareness of Wong's line drawings mirror her blunted senses and the exhaustion from which she cannot escape, as her psychological world is figuratively drained of detail and colour. Although there are three people in the bedroom, Wong appears to be completely isolated, except for the brief materialization of her husband when he sleepily speaks a few words. In the final panel of the sequence, Wong's own form is composed of merely thirteen or so lines of ink, with two additional lines serving as blanket and pillow, an intensely bare representation that reflects the desolation and severity of her inner world. This last panel is drawn from an overhead point of view, blocking out any possibility of seeing her husband and baby as her thoughts become fully narrowed on her own self-doubt. The accoutrements of sleep – the blanket and pillow – are so useless that they barely exist, and the bed has disappeared altogether.

Elsewhere in the narrative, Wong's Chinese immigrant elders foster a form of family caregiving very different from the mainstream Canadian treatment of new mothers. Wong notes that "in Chinese culture, mom and baby are confined to the house for the first month after birth. The mom gets

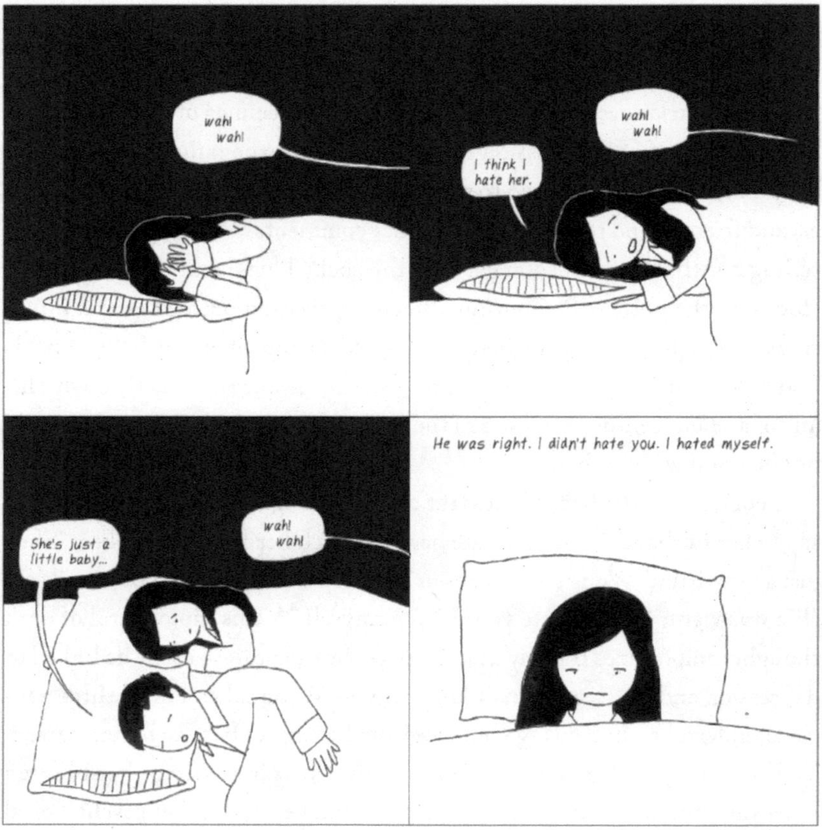
wah! wah!
wah! wah!
I think I hate her.
She's just a little baby...
wah! wah!
He was right. I didn't hate you. I hated myself.

1.1 Teresa Wong, *Dear Scarlet: The Story of My Postpartum Depression* (2019), 73.

a chance to recover while the grandmother gets quality baby time. It is somewhat great, since there is no pressure for new mothers to bounce back quickly. But also somewhat terrible because it can be so isolating."[37] The intermingling of these different cultural traditions allows Wong to assess their respective value systems, and eventually she finds better support both in and out of the home, yet the problems of sleeplessness and depression remain unsolved until an epilogue that traces the later stages of her parenting life.

Problems with sleep often reach their greatest severity as a result of poverty and housing insecurity.[38] Another graphic memoir, *Tower 25* by P.J. Patten of Burnaby, British Columbia, portrays a contemporary experience of homelessness and addiction. When Patten, who was living in his childhood home of Southern California at the time, is evicted from his condo and has

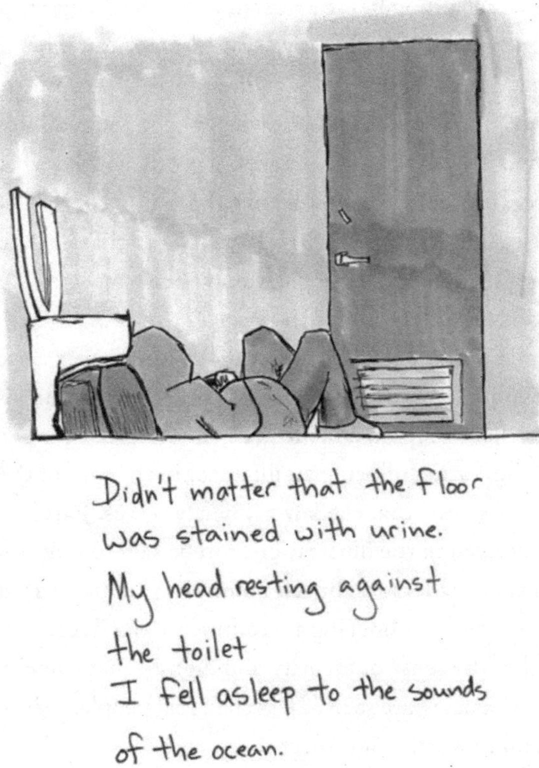
Didn't matter that the floor
was stained with urine.
My head resting against
the toilet
I fell asleep to the sounds
of the ocean.

1.2 P.J. Patten, *Tower 25* (2020), 29.

nowhere else to go, the first problem that arises is the matter of "trying to find a place to sleep."[39] Sleeping overnight in public is illegal, and Patten is woken by the glare of a police flashlight when he is caught sleeping on the ground. "It is against the law to be homeless in many places," he observes.[40] The sleep problem seems intractable for someone who cannot afford an apartment or a hotel; bus stops and picnic tables are too exposed, alleys and parks too dangerous.[41] "Sleep was always stalking me," he writes. "I couldn't escape the exhaustion. I would fall asleep at random whenever I sat down."[42] Eventually, Patten starts sleeping in a public bathroom near a lifeguard tower, Tower 25, on Huntington Beach south of Los Angeles. "It was small, smelled like piss," he says, "but there was a toilet & a door that locked."[43] In these conditions, while falling increasingly ill from exposure, he contemplates the origins of his homelessness, including being arrested at age fourteen for a suicide attempt, after which the criminal justice system accelerated his descent into methamphetamine addiction.[44] After eight months of sleeping in the public bathroom, Patten finally sees a way out when he is accepted into a Buddhist monastery, although even this opportunity is nearly dashed when he is once again caught illegally sleeping and ordered to appear in court.[45] Commenting on his approach to illustrating the story, Patten notes that he "kept the drawings faceless with the hope that people would see themselves, someone they knew, or strangers on the street in these pages."[46]

The criminalization of sleep is an indignity that never arises as a concern for those who have access to housing. Only the most debased form of sleep – a restless half-sleep on a urine-stained concrete floor – is subjected to the further humiliation of being an illicit act in the eyes of the law and of the housing-secure public that the law primarily serves. Patten's decision to keep his face concealed in the illustrations can be said to reflect not only the hopeful notion that readers might see themselves in his situation but also the fact that people without housing are routinely denied recognition of their personhood and of the sense of identity and dignity that comes with it. Just as people without housing are seen as less than real people, their sleep is seen as illegitimate and unworthy of respect.[47]

As part of her 2014 study on the politics of time, media and cultural studies professor Sarah Sharma went to the downtown branch of the Vancouver Public Library "nearly every weekday morning for a month," carefully observing the comings and goings of library patrons.[48] Her observations show that the problem of sleep as an illicit act for those without housing in Vancouver closely echoes Patten's experience in California. By the time the library opens at 10:00 a.m. each morning, nearly a hundred homeless people, mostly men, are lined up waiting to enter. When the security guard opens the door, the people rush inside to their routine places – desks, computer terminals, and private carousels among the book stacks – where they surreptitiously fall asleep. "The city's homeless have come to the library to sleep," Sharma writes. "But they sleep under the guise of other activities because sleeping in the public library is not allowed." The sleepers arrange towers of books on tables to hide their faces from view, or they learn to sleep sitting perfectly upright with one hand on a computer mouse. "The guards know the sleepers," Sharma explains, "and the guards know what the sleepers are doing. But if these tired souls *appear* to be spending their library time wisely, they will not be asked to leave ... The unstated order is about a moral use of time oriented around being productive."

The sleep that is on offer in the library is surely a broken and uncomfortable sleep, yet the patrons have been waiting all night to get it. The alternative would be an even more socially unacceptable sleep, along the lines of Patten's bathroom sleep, that draws the attention of the police with their flashlights and court summonses. This reality makes the public library a deeply ambivalent place that highlights the social expectations around whose sleep can be respected. Sharma notes that, as a refuge for members of the homeless population, the library is "a progressive space,"[49] yet the library must officially deny the legitimacy of the sleep that it quietly permits. The library is in a very difficult position; it is not meant to serve as a hostel, yet its status as a public facility with a social mission calls for a certain degree of flexibility in allowing those without beds to get some rest. As a result, the library is also a place where those who are bedless intermingle with those who are housing-secure, and the power imbalance between the two groups is apparent in the fact that the members of the one must sleep in full view of the members of the other. Having one's sleep exposed to the view of another is a form of vulnerability and intimacy that the more privileged members of society can keep confined to the privacy of their own homes. The situation also means that those who visit the library to read a book or use a computer may find themselves having the uncomfortable feeling that they are intruding on the sleep of others. These patrons must revise their own understanding of sleep by accepting that it is okay for them to walk and read among the sleepers, or they must make an uneasy judgment about which group of people – the readers or the sleepers – has the more legitimate claim to the space. Meanwhile, caught in the middle, the librarians find themselves suffering from burnout since they are compelled to act as untrained social workers.[50]

For those members of society who have access to a more secure sleep environment – a private bedroom at home, maybe with a luxury mattress and an aromatherapy diffuser – a massive economic infrastructure exists to support good sleep, an arrangement that frames sleep not merely as a bodily act but also as a marketable product and an engine of profit and efficiency. Nap It Up is a power nap studio in Toronto where exhausted business workers can pay to take a nap in the middle of the workday. Using the tagline "Recharge

Yourself," Nap It Up promises that power naps of specific durations can boost performance, alertness, or creativity.[51] Clients can pay extra for anti-snoring nose strips and white noise machines. Aside from the questionable promises – Does a fifty-five-minute nap session really improve short-term memory specifically? What if the client needs twenty of these minutes just to fall asleep? – the notion of a daytime nap for tired members of the public makes for an illuminating comparison with the sleepers at the library. If you have money, a daytime sleep makes you a productive go-getter rather than a burden on society.[52]

This framing of sleep as an instrument of productivity is not limited to the consumer sleep market but also makes its way into medical sleep clinics. The Centre for Sleep and Human Performance in Calgary is a sleep lab, testing, and therapy facility for treating a wide variety of sleep disorders.[53] Such clinics can be vitally important for those suffering from sleep apnea, insomnia, and other conditions, yet as its name suggests, the clinic tends to frame sleep in the service of the culture of productivity. The lab's medical director, Dr Charles Samuels, promotes the "strategic" use of sleep and caffeine in order to remedy not only the feeling of fatigue but also the "lack of performance and poor concentration."[54] This use of sleep raises questions about who and what sleep is *for*. Is sleep something we do to increase our value within the economic system? To better achieve our personal life goals? To feel more alert? Or does sleep have intrinsic value regardless of any notions of performance and productivity? The question of why we go to sleep each night is more profound than it may appear, being closely tied to the question of what it means to lead a good life. As I discuss below, such concerns arise not only during visits to specialty sleep clinics but also through mundane acts such as watching mattress ads.

This merely scratches the surface of the cultures of sleep in Canada, but what these examples reveal is that sleep as a universal human act cannot be separated from its political dimensions and that sleep takes shape in this nation in diverse and inequitable ways. Pierre Trudeau famously said that "there's no place for the state in the bedrooms of the nation," yet the values, meanings, and historical legacies that form Canadian cultural life have always intruded into people's most intimate sleeping quarters.[55] The ideologies of the social world are already waiting for you in bed when you climb under the covers (to say nothing of when you lie down on a bench at a transit terminal), and the particular way that these ideologies affect you depends in large part on your position within systemic structures of privilege and power.

It is no wonder, then, that images of sleep, that most harmless of activities, can spark controversy and anger and that representations of sleep in cultural texts of all kinds, from phone apps to experimental poetry, can clarify, question, and even shape the contested roles that sleep plays within the public realm. Indeed, the cases discussed above all involve a combination of actual sleep and the representation of sleep. This is true not just for the published memoirs but also for the incident of the men on the bench whose sleep became the subject of photographs and news articles, for Sharma's narrative about watching sleepers at the library, for the branding of naps as a way to "Recharge Yourself," and even for the statistics arranged in charts by age and gender. We encounter sleep not just as an act but also as an object of representation and discourse, meaning that sleep is part of, not separate from, the ideologies of waking life. Sleep can carry a sense of danger and uncertainty within the public sphere because it is tied culturally to questions of whose voices and representations are seen and heard.

Consider the case of a series of billboards installed in Vancouver as part of the 2021 Capture Photography Festival. Each billboard displayed a photographic portrait of a sleeping person presented by local artist Steven Shearer. Rather than conveying a sense of peaceful slumber, however, the subjects of the photos appeared slovenly and alarmingly unconscious. A topless man on his back, shot from directly above, lies awkwardly on dead grass, his arm bent painfully under his body. A comatose woman slumps in the back seat of a car, her neck uncomfortably bent and her mouth hanging open. The photos create the impression that they have been taken without the subjects' knowledge or consent by a photographer who should have instead been calling for a paramedic. The billboard campaign immediately sparked "various complaints including that the images were of deceased subjects, that they were frightening, and that they evoked the opioid and the homelessness crises."[56] Under intense public pressure, the advertising agency covered up the billboards within two days. This decision, in turn, led to even more media coverage and public commentary, with some expressing outrage at the inappropriate photos and others, such as urban planner Gordon Harris in a *Globe and Mail* opinion piece, accusing small-minded Vancouverites of unconscionable censorship.[57]

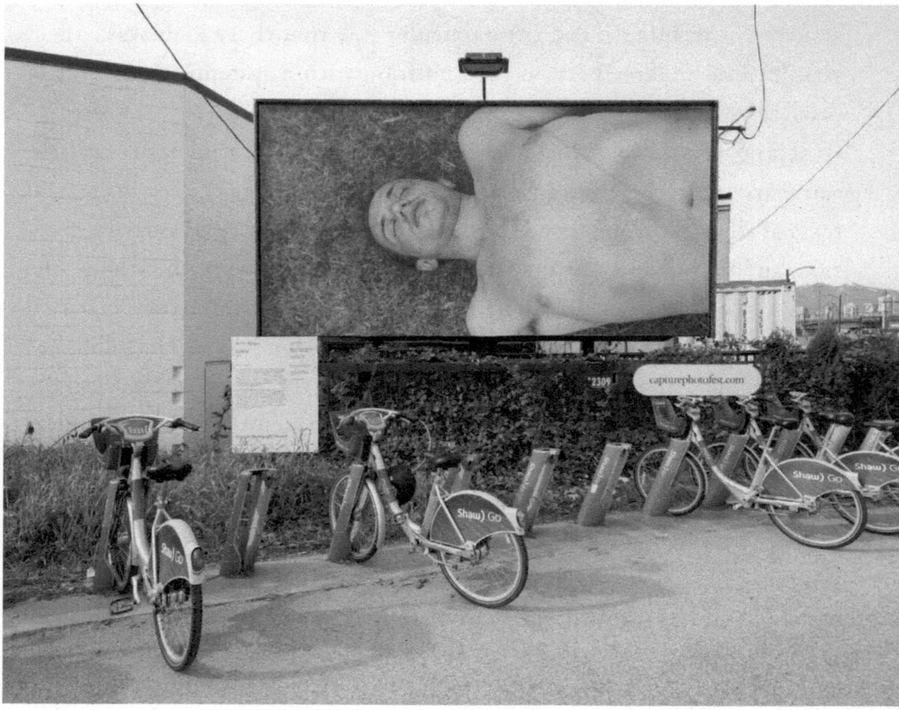

1.3 Steven Shearer, *Untitled* (detail), 2020.

The festival's executive director, Emmy Lee Wall, defended the photographs, arguing that they "offer a provocative and public commentary on the ways in which banal moments are often shared for public consumption" and that the public's complaints represented "a confirmation that these works functioned as was curatorially intended by sparking a dialogue about the thin line between public and private in contemporary society."[58] She further argued that some of the images should be understood as "echoing the poses found in religious paintings and sculptures wherein the bodies appear to be in states of ecstasy or defying gravity, released from their earthly bonds."[59] This may be a bit of a stretch, although visual art scholar Catherine Heard agrees that the pose of a sleeping person draped in fabric on one of the festival billboards bears a resemblance to Gian Lorenzo Bernini's 1652 sculpture *Ecstasy of Saint Teresa*, and for her, the photo of the man on the grass brings to mind Giuseppe Sanmartino's 1753 sculpture *The Veiled Christ*. Arguing that "context is everything in interpreting images," Heard notes that viewers of *The Veiled Christ* in the Sansevero Chapel Museum in Naples will find that their interpretation "is shaped both by the Christian religious context established by the chapel museum, and by the sculpture's central position in the building ... By comparison, the low materiality and association of the snapshot as a throw-away image frames Shearer's sleepers as abject bodies, flawed and vulnerable in their unconscious state. Their gestures can equally be read as ungainly."[60]

If the photo series can be said to raise critical questions about the public face of sleep, we might say that the billboards brought to light the normative values that govern what kind of sleep is acceptable, namely the idea that sleep, especially when put on display for public consumption, should look peaceful, not frightening. The vulnerability of sleep should reflect innocence and safety while reinforcing acceptable sleeping places such as bedrooms; it should not reflect ugliness, slovenliness, and the shameful use of inappropriate sleeping places such as fields of dying grass. If sleep must be public, it is okay for the sleeper to be tousled but not repulsive. When sleepers are ugly and sleeping in the wrong place (or when their sleep is displayed in the wrong place), sleep no longer reflects peaceful innocence; it now reflects the horrors and bitter politics of the waking world with its crises of opioid use and homelessness. Mixed in with these concerns is the matter of consent, which the subjects of the photos were not able to grant when the images were captured and, it turns out, did not grant for the billboard installation at all. Shearer did not take the photos himself but selected them from a collection of "found" images "mined from the internet, eBay and various print media."[61] For the festival curators, the strange life course of these photos, from private snapshots to instigators of moral panic, was not an embarrassment but an important feature that helped to spark provocative public dialogue.

However all of these factors may be construed, the complaints about the photos being alarming were quite unsurprising. Any dialogue that the billboards may have sparked about the public consumption of private moments or about representations of the sacred and the profane was likely confined to the scholars, curators, and media commentators who had insight into the context of the photo series and its artistic ambitions. A viewer who was unarmed with a copy of the exhibit catalogue (or, quite understandably, did not notice or absorb the smaller information panels below the enormous, disturbing billboards) would have been hard-pressed to say whether the subjects depicted were alive or dead, a fact that could not have been lost on the festival directors. The images could have been foreseen as being likely to disturb the public, and in this sense the installation can be understood not as a critical commentary on representations of sleep but as a manipulation of the ambiguities of the sleeping human form to create unnecessary controversy and raise a commotion about the photo festival. The case of the billboards shows how sleep, in its capacity as a subject of representation, is a complex site of cultural politics that can be made to serve different agendas. Sleep is a locus of normative values, a fulcrum for social critique, and a potent, potentially cynical tool for the manipulation of public discourse. Sometimes representations of sleep raise critical questions about how we conceive of sleep, and sometimes they are not really about sleep at all.

Another illuminating and uneasy representation of sleep comes from filmmaker and visual artist Shelley Niro, a Turtle Clan member from the Six Nations Reserve.[62] As I discuss again in later chapters, sleep often has a particular vitality for Indigenous Peoples, especially in terms of the sacredness of dreams, and Indigenous writers such as Willie Ermine have identified important connections between dreaming and the cultural structures of identity and knowledge.[63] However, as noted earlier, sleep has also served as a form of oppression through colonization, as in the use of inadequate sleeping arrangements in residential schools. Likewise, Benjamin Reiss notes that colonial rule has often involved attempts by European authorities to deem Indigenous sleeping arrangements "perverse" and to eradicate them.[64] The denigration of Indigenous Peoples through the stereotype of the "lazy Indian," meanwhile, constitutes a violent deployment of the notion of sleep. For Indigenous artists, these contested visions allow sleep to serve as a figure of cultural strength or as a figure of resistance and irony.

Sleeping Warrior, Dressing Warrior is a collage by Niro that offers an ironic response to the colonial notions that have been imposed on Indigenous Peoples. At the centre of the collage is an Indigenous man, the warrior, who appears confidently at home sleeping on a blanket draped carelessly over an ornate chaise longue. Naked, except for a pair of moccasin slippers, an embroidered satchel, a feather, and some fabric placed over his groin, the warrior sleeps with one hand behind his head and one foot trailing on the floor. Positioned around him, taking up the bulk of the collage, is a collection of outfits and accessories for a paper dress-up doll that are perfectly suited to his

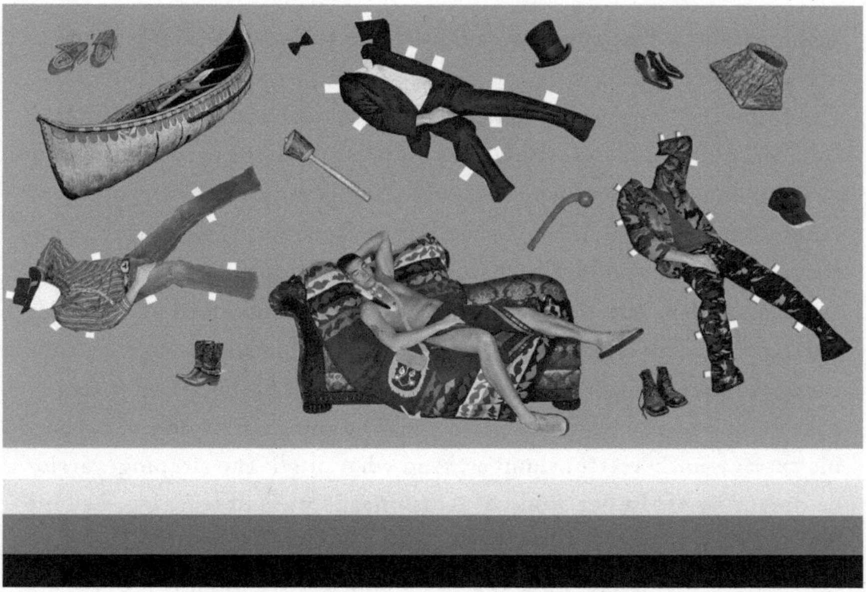

1.4 Shelley Niro, *Sleeping Warrior, Dressing Warrior*, 2012.

size and posture. Viewers are thus invited to cut out the clothes and dress the sleeping warrior however they like – in camo fatigues, a tuxedo, or a cowboy outfit – or they can leave his default near-nudity untouched. Accessories for the warrior include a top hat, a baseball cap, and a canoe. That the warrior sleeps through this situation and does not resist implicitly endorses the dismissal of his agency through the structure of the dress-up game.

The arrangement of this collage, where the viewer is granted an uncomfortable degree of power over the sleeping man, mimics the way that the colonizing society has often imposed certain traits and characteristics on Indigenous Peoples while denying their agency and their right to self-definition. The viewer of the collage will never see the Indigenous man – figured here in a way that may conjure the "lazy Indian" stereotype – as a conscious subject in his own right. By making this power dynamic so blatant, the collage satirizes the audacity of the colonizing society in presuming to see Indigenous people as less than human, as playthings or cardboard cut-outs to be manipulated at will. Although the collage is ostensibly designed to be used as a dress-up set, viewers are likely to feel a sense of unease at the thought of actually dressing and undressing the sleeping man

– an uneasiness that may also cause them to reflect on the larger context of the colonizing gaze.

Meanwhile, the sleeping warrior holds a subtle but important degree of confidence and power. Not only does his presence in the dress-up set bring about a canny satire on colonial visions of Indigeneity, but his unconcerned pose also suggests that he has found a way to rise above (by sleeping through) the troubles of his politically charged dress-up world. Moreover, there is a sense in which he effortlessly reverses the direction of colonial power; while the trappings of colonization swirl around him, he himself has colonized the European chaise longue by draping his blanket and his body over it, its elegant frame and ornately patterned gold fabric now existing only to support his extravagantly restful slumber. And what might the sleeping warrior be dreaming of? In her study of Anishinaabe ways of learning, Leanne Betasamosake Simpson writes that "knowledge is often transmitted from the spiritual world to humans through dreaming and visioning."[65] The dreams of the sleeping warrior may be a fount of cultural power, they may be more mundane, or perhaps he is not dreaming at all. This knowledge belongs only to him, as the colonial gaze cannot penetrate his slumber. The white, yellow, red, and black stripes along the bottom of the image (reproduced here in black and white) call to mind the form of a national flag and the colours of the medicine wheel, making the sleeping warrior, both earnestly and mockingly, a distinguished Indigenous icon. Among the things that the warrior is fighting for, we might conclude, is the assertion that a critical literacy of sleep is necessary for comprehending a diverse and unequal cultural world.

"WHAT KEEPS YOU AWAKE?": TRAVELLING TO SLEEP COUNTRY

Cultural texts and practices in Canada thus cast light on the representations of sleep particular to this country. This is not to say that there is a singular "Canadian" vision of sleep but rather that multiple visions collectively make up a tangled configuration of values and practices linked to cultures of sleep within a diverse nation. To be sure, cultural representations of sleep circulate across borders; an infamous tweet by the American company Netflix, for instance, that "Sleep is my greatest enemy"[66] certainly reverberated beyond the

United States. Even though the tweet takes a humorous tone in advocating nighttime binge-watching, its sentiment is typical of the tendency of capitalism to discourage sleep (restful slumber being so difficult to monetize), and the appeal to wakeful consumption finds echoes in many parts of the world. Nevertheless, uncovering the nuances of diverse representations particular to Canada reveals that sleep is deployed in this nation for multiple purposes founded on allegiances to competing values. In the final section of this chapter, rather than looking at overtly negative representations of sleep, I look at a cluster of texts that appear to support and celebrate sleep. On close examination, texts that encourage good sleep are often not as divorced as they might seem from the notion that sleep is an enemy to overcome. Learning how to recognize the contradictions of sleep-positive texts is a key element in building a literacy of sleep, and this skill can lead us toward more creative visions of what it might mean to approach sleep with curiosity and respect.

One of the most visible homes of sleep as a cultural figure in this nation is Sleep Country Canada, the mattress and bedding supply retailer founded in 1994 and now operating stores across nearly all provinces. The company's advertisements are well known, particularly the earlier ads featuring co-founder Christine Magee and the company's signature jingle. Their website declares that "Sleep Country is Canada's leading specialty retailer dedicated to sleep ... With all things for all sleepers, we can help you get a better night's sleep."[67] Sara Arber and her collaborators are among those who have observed that sleep has become a consumer good,[68] and indeed, as is often the case in the sleep product industry, Sleep Country Canada positions itself less as a purveyor of mattresses than of sleep itself. The firm's ticker symbol on the Toronto Stock Exchange is ZZZ.

Sleep Country's more recent advertising campaigns, which feature increasingly polished cinematography, develop a complex series of associations linking mattresses and other sleep products with two central needs, or deficiencies, presumed to exist in the audience: the need to alleviate the problems that cause sleep loss and the need to enable daytime productivity. I look at three ads in particular to tease apart the nuances of the work that sleep is being made to do. The first two ads develop a narrative about addressing the problem of insomnia, but although the ads seemingly take the sources of insomnia as their focus, a recognition of the systemic causes of sleep loss is always deferred. This evasiveness allows the ads to remain within the safer realm of the particular sleep troubles that can be solved by mattresses and duvets. Viewers of these ads are thus validated by having their sleep loss recognized, but they are also left in isolation and perhaps in shame if they happen to suffer from sleep problems, whether systemic or individual, that fall outside those that Sleep Country can solve. In the third ad, the figure of sleep enables a critique of social acceleration and the culture of overwork, yet this critique is inevitably compromised by conflicting values, as the desirability of a good mattress in a sense requires the perpetuation of a culture of exhaustion. Sleep can therefore be said to operate both as the antidote to and as the enabler of the insomniac 24/7 society.

"What Keeps You Awake?" is one of a series of Sleep Country ads that catalogue the various problems that prevent people from sleeping.[69] Company president Christine Magee opens the ad by asking the camera, "What keeps you awake at night?" In response, a sequence of shots portrays customers explaining the sources of their sleep loss. A woman points to her husband and says, "Mr Restless over there keeps waking me up." A different man appears and says simply, "A sore back." He is followed by a man who complains, "I'm too hot," earning a frown from his female companion who says, "I'm too cold." The ad then shifts to shots of these customers and others enjoying their new mattresses, while Magee returns in the form of a voiceover and says, "Sleep Country has the best beds for every sleep problem and budget." Other similar ads in this series focus on aches, pains, and night sweats.

The central promise of the ads is that the right mattress can solve "every sleep problem," yet the only problems mentioned are forms of physical discomfort. Left unspoken are the many other prevalent causes of sleeplessness, ranging from the behavioural to the systemic, which include demanding work schedules, caffeine, alcohol, poverty, the inequities of gendered labour, and – at the top of the list for many people – anxiety and worry.[70] Comfortable as they may be, mattresses and pillows cannot solve most of these quandaries. Because the company must avoid raising any problems their sleep products cannot address, the advertisements must sweep under the rug some of the behavioural issues that prevent good sleep and, most especially, the cultural sources of insomnia that plague society.

Interestingly, one Sleep Country ad broaches the subject of anxiety, flirting dangerously with the societal and psychological problems that, if acknowledged, would highlight the limitations of retail sleep products. "Turn

Off the Lights. And Your Brain" is an ad whose protagonist, a young woman, spends a torturous night in bed staring at the ceiling.[71] While she fidgets with the blankets, frustration and concern written on her face, her own voiceover provides commentary, the pacing of which starts out slow and then rapidly accelerates in panic: "So I'm lying in bed unable to get comfy, and then I think, 'Oh no, I can't sleep,' which makes it impossible to sleep, and then tomorrow there'll be all this pressure to sleep, which means I can't sleep again, and then after three weeks of not sleeping my immune system will fail, and I'll burst a blood vessel in my eye." The scene then changes to a Sleep Country retail store, where a sales rep who has been listening to this anguished explanation reassures the woman: "Don't worry – you've come to the right place. We have lots of comfy beds for you to choose from." In the final shot, the woman sleeps soundly on her new bed.

The true source of the protagonist's insomnia is ambiguous. Her self-diagnosis, that she is "unable to get comfy," sets up the sales rep's pitch for comfortable beds, yet the customer's extended narrative reveals that she is unable to sleep because she is worried about not being able to sleep, a problem that the ad can only address at a slant angle. The notion that better comfort will address her problem is somewhat plausible but too optimistic, and the logical leap that identifies uncomfortable bedding as the source of her anxiety becomes very fragile under scrutiny. This sense of self-deception within the sleep industry and its customers has sometimes been the target of keenly perceptive ridicule, such as in a headline from the satirical online newspaper *The Onion*: "Weighted Blanket Sure to Succeed Where CBD, Salt Lamp, Oil Diffuser, Acupressure Mat, Bath Bombs, and White Noise Machine Failed."[72] No amount of relaxing bedroom accessories (or bothersome, distracting accessories, for that matter) can stop the insomniac from staring, terrified and shattered, into the abyss.

Whereas "What Keeps You Awake?" silently omits anxiety from the list of problems that cause insomnia, "Turn Off the Lights" boldly focuses on the anxious worrying of its protagonist, and the ad thus comes perilously close to acknowledging the reality that insomnia often cannot be solved by a mattress. The ad therefore reaches, and defines, the analytical limit that Sleep Country is unable to cross. In creeping closer to a comprehensive vision of the sources of sleep loss – moving from hot bedrooms and restless partners to the profound terrors of anxiety – these ads offer a sense of solidarity and support for the sleepless, but they stop short of pinpointing, and indeed must skirt and suppress, the cultural and psychological problems at the heart of widespread insomnia in the modern world. In this way, the community of belonging to which consumer sleep products give shape is shadowed by a hinterland of systemic sleeplessness that remains unspoken and thus delegitimized.

"SLEEP IS FOR THE STRONG"

"Sleep Is for the Strong," released in 2017, is the Sleep Country ad that I want to focus on most closely due to its rich implications for understanding popular cultures of sleep.[73] Set to upbeat music, and unexpectedly fast-paced for a sleep product commercial, the thirty-second ad rapidly depicts two days in the life of a young, white, male corporate office worker who is overwhelmed by the demands of productivity and the fast pace of working life. He is so exhausted and rushed that he walks straight into a glass wall while looking at his phone. He spills coffee on his lap while looking too quickly at his watch. Files and documents are stacked so high on his desk that they collapse and topple to the ground. A voiceover says, "You grind and you grind. Deadline after deadline. Show up early, stay latest, work harder, be the greatest. Meeting at 8 p.m., then 8 a.m. ASAP, ETA, TBD, with no time for Zs." The employee and his co-workers struggle to stay awake during the 8:00 p.m. meeting, pens in hands and cups of coffee on the table. Following this meeting, a quick shot of a clock with a rapidly swinging second hand fades from 8:00 p.m. to 8:00 a.m., the two identical clock times distinguishable from one another only because of a change in lighting as night transitions to day. The worker is now seated, exhausted as ever, in the 8:00 a.m. meeting that has taken the place of the 8:00 p.m. meeting. Like the times on the clock, the two meetings are nearly indistinguishable, with only the slightest differences making the second day distinct from the first; a dark-blue collared shirt now peeks out from under the worker's light-grey sweater, replacing the light-blue collared shirt and light-blue sweater of the previous day.

As darkness falls in the office, the worker makes his way to the bus stop, where he immediately falls asleep on the bench, toppling over in a manner reminiscent of his stack of documents. When he arrives home, he is excited to see a large box marked "Bloom" waiting outside his door. The voiceover

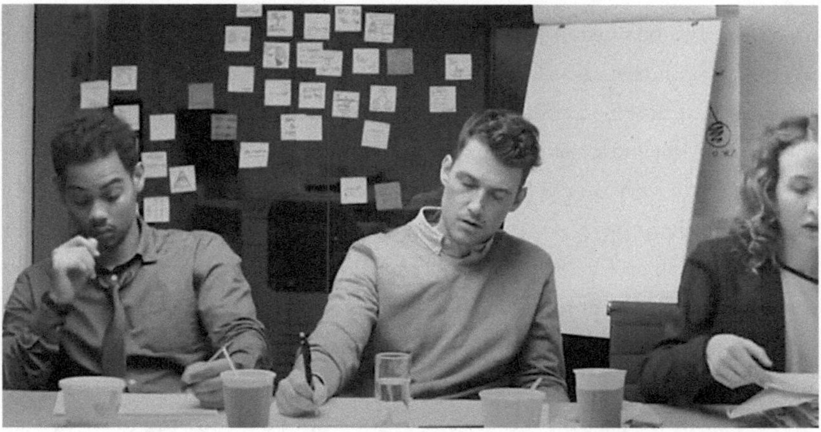

1.5 Sleep Country Canada, "#SleepIsForTheStrong – Introducing Sleep Country's Bloom™ Mattress in a Box," 2017.

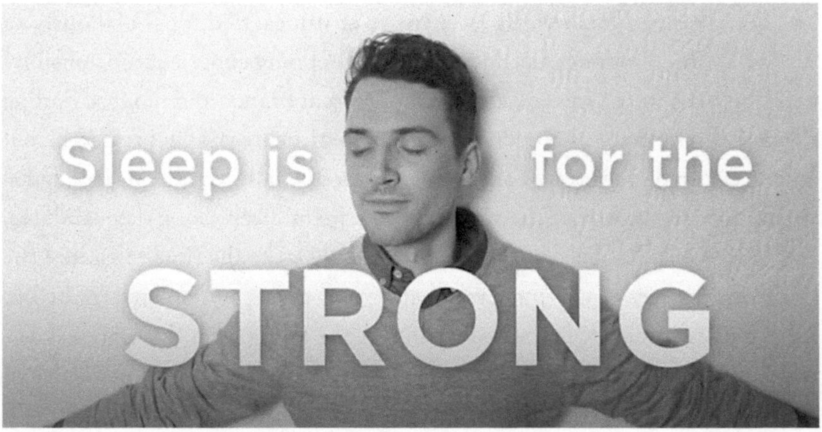

1.6 Sleep Country Canada, "#SleepIsForTheStrong – Introducing Sleep Country's Bloom™ Mattress in a Box," 2017.

states, "'Sleep is for the weak,' they say. No way. Sleep is for the strong. Bloom. By Sleep Country." Inside his apartment, the worker pulls out the Bloom mattress, collapses onto it, and enters a blissful sleep, still wearing his office attire and dress shoes. The tagline appears over his slumbering form: "Sleep is for the STRONG."

Given that the Sleep Country brand is heavily associated with traditional retail stores, their Bloom product line serves to compete in the growing online mattress sales business – known as the "mattress in a box" category – popularized by brands such as Casper and Endy (the latter of which was acquired by Sleep Country in 2018). Aimed primarily at young adults who prefer to shop online, the mattress in a box model ostensibly makes the process of buying a mattress very quick; the customer selects from a few standard models online, and then the mattress arrives at their door rolled up in a box. "All you need to do," Sleep Country explains in their written description, "is unbox the mattress, let it 'bloom,' and start dreaming."[74] Literary scholar Hilary Hinds has shown that the choice of a bed is not merely a matter of comfort and price but reflects shifting cultural visions of family relationships and other values. She focuses on the history of the twin bed, showing how the rise of twin beds for married couples in Britain starting in the late nineteenth century, and their decline in the second half of the twentieth century, reflected and shaped changing notions of "hygiene, modernity and marriage."[75] The mattress in a box reveals its own set of values, tied most obviously to the fast online shopping method. I call the shopping experience "ostensibly" quick because the process of comparing different brands and models, finding the best promotions, and trying to sort out legitimate product reviews from fake ones can be very time-consuming. In theory, however, the near-magical appearance of the box at the worker's apartment after a long day validates, and indeed enables, his frantic life, as he clearly lacks the time to endure the laborious process of visiting a retail store and trying out a mattress before buying it. A second value rolled up in the box along with the mattress is a reliance on ecologically costly supply chains, a problem that is pervasive in online shopping but is omitted from the ad.[76]

"Sleep Is for the Strong" apparently intends to promote the importance of good sleep, but its position as a sleep-positive text is fraught with contradictions. The ambivalence of the ad hinges on the fact that it portrays the primary function of sleep as enabling frantic, pointless work. The worker suffers from exhaustion because his job is unreasonably demanding; he therefore rewards himself with a new mattress that will replenish his energy so that he can continue to perform well in his job, thus further exhausting himself. In this way, the ad reflects the assertion by Arber and her collaborators that constant busyness has become a status symbol in Western societies, leading to a devaluation of sleep, with the result that sleep tends to be promoted and celebrated only to serve the goal of increasing work efficiency.[77] An emphasis on the importance of good sleep can be said to normalize and support a culture of overwork.

A similar notion has often emerged in critical studies of time. In his study of social acceleration, sociologist Hartmut Rosa observes that attempts to resist the exhausting fast pace of modern life often have a counterintuitive effect, ultimately exacerbating the frenetic culture of speed. Yoga classes, for example, may be presented as a way to slow down, a way to counteract the exhaustion of social acceleration, but by replenishing the energy reserves of the participants, yoga can effectively "serve the goal of coping with the swift-paced life of the workplace."[78] Slowing down thus becomes a strategy of acceleration, and in this sense yoga serves a similar purpose to the coffee break: a momentary pause through which the participants inject energy into their bloodstream. Media and cultural studies scholar Sarah Sharma, who studies diverse and inequitable forms of time use, has developed important rebuttals to many generalizations about the accelerating pace of life, but on this matter she reaches similar conclusions to Rosa. She argues that initiatives such as yoga classes, by making it easier for people to cope with overwork, might drain people of their motivation to support labour activism, with the result that "yoga at work may make a shorter workweek harder to fight for."[79] Sure enough, as the worker in the Sleep Country ad falls asleep with a very slight smile on his face, he appears ready to jump right back into action, living up to the demands of his workplace without any need to fight for systemic change.

Other ads posted on Sleep Country's social media channels, using the tagline "Sleep is the fuel that powers your day," further emphasize the idea that the purpose of sleep is to enable daytime productivity.[80] Using both the fuel metaphor and a charging battery metaphor to convey the notion of abundant energy, these ads show people not enjoying a restful sleep but waking up and stretching their freshly charged bodies. Sleep, much like electricity or gasoline, is an energy resource to be accumulated and spent in the service of exuberant activity. In their analysis of popular sleep-tracking apps and gadgets, Diletta De Cristofaro and Simona Chiodo note that quantitative sleep measurements "are reshaping our sense of self," causing their users to obsessively evaluate their own existence through calculations of personal achievement.[81] Sleep-tracking technologies, they argue, "can be interpreted as the tools through which achievement-subjects work on improving themselves as their own entrepreneurial projects."[82] The social media ads from

Sleep Country suggest that the compulsion to become an "achievement-subject" is reinforced not only by products that use quantification but even by those that advance a more qualitative vision of replenishment. Promoting a sales event called "Better Sleep, Better You," one Sleep Country ad promises that you will be able to "run farther" after a good sleep.[83] The focus here is not on measuring the distance of the run per se but on the feeling of being energized, of being ready to achieve better things. By shifting the focus from the sleeping body to the powered-up body, these ads show that Sleep Country is in the business of selling wakefulness. Yes, when you arrive in Sleep Country, you will have a good sleep, but more importantly you will then leave sleep behind with energy to burn.

Getting back to "Sleep Is for the Strong," another key element of the ad is that by emphasizing the notion of strength, the tagline apparently subverts the popular assertion, often used half-jokingly, that "sleep is for the weak." Although these two statements seemingly take opposite positions, they ultimately reflect a surprisingly compatible vision of sleep and strength. For instance, the notion of strength in the sense of resilience and endurance is central to the use of the phrase "sleep is for the weak" in the genre of semi-ironic motherhood support writing. Several books in this genre use the phrase in their title, such as Amy Eschliman and Leigh Oshirak's *Balance Is a Crock, Sleep Is for the Weak: An Indispensable Guide to Surviving Working Motherhood*, Rita Arens's *Sleep Is for the Weak: The Best of the Mommybloggers*, and Emily-Jane Clark's *Sleep Is for the Weak: How to Survive When Your Baby Won't Go the F**k to Sleep*. The phrase here takes an ironic tone in the hope that mothers will find humour in their own exhaustion, even while it supports the marketing of the books as parenting aids for women, presenting sleep deprivation as an inevitability that must be endured. The phrase develops a sense of community and solidarity, and the notion of sleep being for the weak actually serves as an assertion of strength in the face of exhausting cultural labour expectations tied to gender, as the demands of parenting are placed primarily on women.

The Sleep Country ad appears to subvert this notion by reclaiming sleep, positioning sleep as a source or characteristic of strength rather than as a luxury or a concession that strong people can get by without. However, the fundamental feature of the worker's strength in the ad, the reason that he is strong, is not that he sleeps but that he uses sleep effectively to maintain his

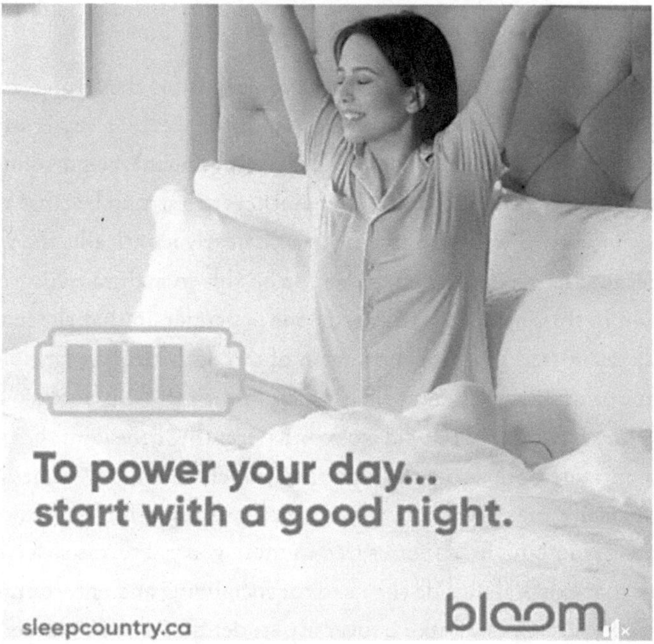

1.7 Sleep Country Canada, "To Power Your Day ... Start with a Good Night," 2020.

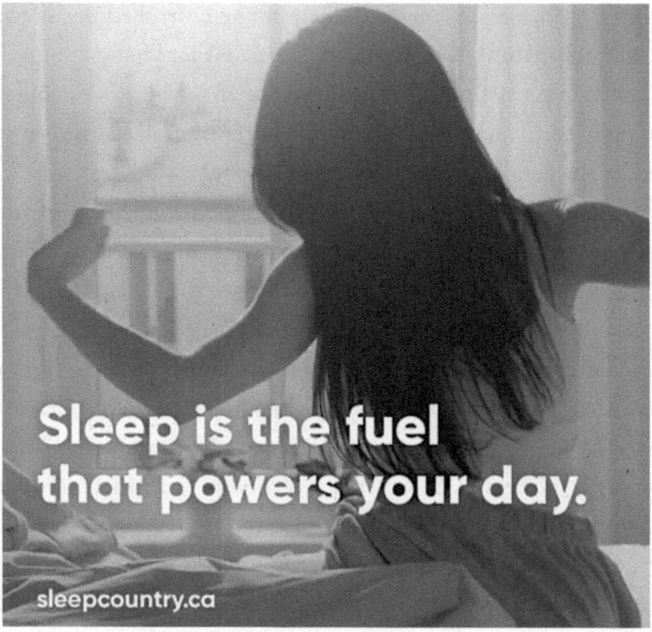

1.8 Sleep Country Canada, "Sleep Is the Fuel That Powers Your Day," 2020.

exhausting work schedule. In other words, "sleep is for the strong" turns out to enforce the same proposition as "sleep is for the weak": sleep is an activity to be resorted to only insofar as it keeps fuelling the merry-go-round of the exhausting frenzy of modern life. The mothers are strong because they can accomplish their work on minimal sleep, and nearly identically, the worker is strong because he gets just enough sleep to be able to maintain his work. The distinction in this instance is primarily one of gender, in that the male office worker is permitted to claim the notion of strength because he holds a job in an important office, whereas the women in the self-help books who must simultaneously endure both paid work and parenting can claim the notion of strength only surreptitiously through their efforts to avoid weakness.

Sexism is not the only factor, as the idea that sleep is for the weak is often used to justify late-night activities tied in more general terms to a culture of overwork that exists alongside the needs of socializing and entertainment. In an editorial for *Huffpost*, Duke University student Carly Stern describes the phrase "sleep is for the weak" as "the college mantra," founded on the premise that "between sleep, good grades and a social life, college students must pick two and cut their losses on the third ... Sleep feels like the most dispensable of the three."[84] The phrase is thus a lament for an overscheduled life as well as an assertion of capability and strength. Sleep loss for young adults in college may be less likely to operate on gendered terms, whereas for older adults wrapped up in the demands of careers and parenting, sleep loss is increasingly shaped by the gendered expectations of labour.[85]

Tied up in these representations is a problematic vision of resilience. Resilience is typically seen in its positive sense as something to aspire to, as a learned skill as well as an inner strength built into the human body. However, resilience can play a worrying role when it caters to a neoliberal vision of the world as a place where all individuals have a personal responsibility to manage their energy reserves in order to facilitate the culture of exhaustion. We might note Tricia Hersey's argument, in *Rest Is Resistance*, that "this culture does not want you rested unless it is attached to your increased labor and productivity ... A large part of your unraveling from capitalism will include becoming less attached to the idea of productivity and more committed to the idea of rest as a portal to just be."[86] Sadly, in the case of the Bloom ad, Hersey's book is not among the documents on the office worker's desk, and although the mattress apparently invites him into a restful slumber, he must strategically deploy his sleep-fuelled resilience in the service of frantic productivity. Indeed, the ad is ambiguous about whether the new mattress will actually allow him to get more sleep or whether it will instead allow him to obtain a higher-quality replenishment in the same amount of time – to sleep faster, as it were.[87]

The prospects of the worker dedicating more hours to sleep seem grim, especially since he doesn't have time to get undressed or turn off the lights. After all, his problem in the first place is not that he has an uncomfortable mattress but that he has "no time for Zs." The concluding moment of the ad, when the worker finally sleeps, is shot from directly overhead, placing him vertically on screen as though he is standing up, eroding the distinction between sleep and wakefulness. This shot closely mirrors some of the earlier scenes where the worker struggles to stay awake in meetings, all with the same clothes and the same heavy eyelids. He has been on the verge of falling asleep all day at work and is now on the verge of wakefulness while he sleeps. He embraces sleep in the most minimal way possible – placing his body on the mattress and closing his eyes – the centrality of work to his identity emblematized by the fact that he remains fully dressed, even his hair staying perfectly styled during his slumber. Already in a pose of readiness, all that he has to do is open his eyes, and he will immediately resume his role as a frantic worker. Sleeping life and working life form a continuous blur, and sleep is presented as just one facet of the perpetual labour of modern existence. One notable feature of the ad is that for all the frenzied work that the employee must do during his long days, the job has no visible purpose. We don't know what the people at this company are meant to accomplish, other than attending meetings and stacking documents. The worker's job is exhausting work for the sake of exhausting work, and his mattress will enable him to keep doing it.

This critique may be starting to verge on the comical, and as is often the case, humour points the way to a layer of truth. It would be somewhat absurd to place the burden of proletarian revolution on the shoulders of the exhausted worker and then shame him for not rising to the challenge. He is, after all, very tired. Comfortable sleep is deeply important, not least for people compelled to lead busy lives, and a good mattress might be considered a profoundly sleep-positive text that provides joy and fills a vital need. Simple beds have been in use for at least 77,000 years, with raised frames and mattresses dating back over 5,000 years to ancient Malta and Egypt.[88] Mattresses are not a ruse or a fad, even if some mattresses are more ecologically costly than others and even if their ads stray into decidedly ideological territory. The relief with which the worker collapses onto the bed is very real, and the slight smile on his face when society finally allows him to replenish his energy cannot so easily be dismissed by his failure to fight for systemic change. Labour activism, too, is a burden that would only add to his to-do list. Likewise, it would be too cynical, and somewhat ridiculous, to condemn Sleep Country Canada for failing to dismantle neoliberal capitalism. Their workers, too, lead busy lives running a bedding supply retailer, and truly, they are right that a comfortable mattress can be a godsend. Both the protagonist of the ad and the vision of sleep to which it caters are caught within a culture of exhaustion larger than themselves, and they both hope to make the best of it.

This ambivalence, then, is at the heart of the business of selling sleep: as a product, sleep is both the antidote to and the enabler of the insomniac 24/7 society. Presented as a commodity, sleep can make individual moments within the culture of exhaustion more bearable, a truly valuable proposition. Of all the texts discussed in this book, it is doubtful that any can support good sleep as much as a mattress, a fact that may be obvious but cannot be overlooked. Nevertheless, it is only through imagining sleep differently that the systemic culture of exhaustion can truly be challenged, and for such re-imaginings, we must turn elsewhere. One place in particular where we can identify startling and altogether different visions of sleep is literature.

2

The Poetics of Sleep

AS MATTRESS ADS and other examples reveal, cultural representations of sleep are not merely incidental to the role that sleep plays in society but are intertwined with, and indeed shape, how we imagine and encounter sleep every day. Representations of sleep are illuminating and complex, affecting and cunning, and learning how to read sleep with critical awareness requires the assessment of many different visions of slumber. Literature is one form of representation that can provide thoughtful, nuanced visions of sleep, and if we want to become careful readers of sleep, poetry and fiction are worth our time.

Literature can do two central things for us. It can teach us to see sleep with fresh eyes – to understand and imagine sleep in unexpected ways that reveal the meanings and significance of sleep in diverse contexts. It can also help us develop a critical literacy of sleep by teaching us to notice how sleep operates as a conceptual figure that can push and pull our attention in many directions. Even literature that contemplates drowsiness can foster a sense of alertness, showing us how to identify, question, and when necessary, escape the dominant cultural visions of sleep that circulate around us. In this chapter, I look at how and why literature can seek to represent the experience of sleep, and I examine representations of sleep in poetry from Canada. Although literature of all genres can speak to the complex cultural role of sleep, poetry has a special tendency to engage with elements of language and form in a way that challenges the idea that sleep cannot be directly perceived. In this way, poetry comments on the necessity of literature itself for engaging with sleep. Moving beyond formal experimentation and experiences of sleep, poetry can also use strategies held in common with narrative fiction by developing thematic, philosophical, and political visions of sleep. In so doing, poetry helps to build a larger picture of the contested ways that sleep has been imagined in this nation.

One of the difficulties for those who wish to contemplate sleep is that because it happens outside of what we normally understand as consciousness, sleep cannot easily be represented or even spoken of as a matter of experience. Cressida Heyes notes that "the interruption of self that sleep offers makes it hard to theorize," with the result that philosophical approaches to sleep tend to gloss over the matter of actual sleep, focusing instead on "the surrounding frame in which sleep occurs."[1] This aspect of sleep also creates an acute problem for literature; how can art composed of representation through language engage with something that so slyly resists description? As Benjamin Reiss observes, "Sleep would seem to be resistant to literary treatment, because nothing 'happens' while we sleep, and in a sense we're not even 'there' to have anything happen to us."[2] In his search for works of literature that portray sleep, Reiss points to the literary memoir as a genre that has taken a particular interest in insomnia. For instance, Blake Butler's book *Nothing: A Portrait of Insomnia* speaks of a terrifying period of 129 consecutive sleepless hours endured by the author. Insomnia, however, by definition, is not sleep, and a story about failing to sleep is in a sense the opposite of a story about sleeping. Although Reiss notes that art can portray sleepers as observed by a viewer, he finds that it cannot really portray sleeping itself. "Obviously," he writes, "it's impossible to describe the condition of *being* asleep."[3]

In his book *Sleep and the Novel*, Michael Greaney challenges this view, at least to an extent. Examining the complex representations of sleep in Marcel Proust's *In Search of Lost Time*, Greaney identifies what he calls "the otherness of sleep," which refers to "the sense of sleep as a state in which we are not ourselves, in which the 'I' is temporarily abolished – a plunge into oblivion and absence that seems, paradoxically enough, to be the very condition of the maintenance of a sense of self-sameness over time."[4] Like an asymptotic line that draws closer and closer to the curve that it can never reach, Proust's narrative, by seeking out the experience of sleep, comes ever closer to that inevitable moment when sleep occurs and the possibility of direct experience vanishes. For Greaney, the innovation of Proust's writing comes about largely through "his willingness to dwell intently on, and at, the fringes of sleep,"[5] showing that the ability to narrate the experience of sleep is tantalizingly close but never quite within grasp. Proust might come closer to a narration of sleep than most writers, yet the stubborn truth remains, as Greaney says, that "we can talk *of* sleep but we cannot speak *from* it, and it seems to have nothing to say on its own behalf."[6]

Part of the difficulty here is that, when it comes to sleep, the strengths of narrative fiction also define its limits. A particular aptitude of fiction is its ability to confirm the links between time and identity since the organization of sequential events solidifies the sense of who a person is and how they relate to the world. In his seminal study of time and narrative, Paul Ricoeur asks, "What justifies our taking the subject of an action, so designated by his, her, or its proper name, as the same throughout a life that stretches from birth to death? The answer has to be narrative ... Without the recourse to narration, the problem of personal identity would in fact be condemned to an antinomy with no solution."[7] This is a profoundly useful claim, yet the forms of creativity, memory, and thought that allow us to maintain a narrative identity across time all crucially depend on replenishment through sleep, the very act that escapes the usual bounds of self. Identity may require a sense of narrative, but it also requires us to silence the little narrators in our minds every night. In one of his most memorable aphorisms, Ricoeur observes that "time becomes human time to the extent that it is organized after the manner of a narrative."[8] This account, too, is all very well for the waking world, where personal identity must be made coherent and where time must be made to function in human terms. Sleep, however, confounds personal identity and human time, causing the human subject to evaporate. Thus, although narrative fiction can play a vital role in investigating the peripheries of sleep – the experience of insomnia, the social values attached to sleep, and so on – other forms of representation might be better suited to perceiving sleep from the inside.

In attempting to dissolve personal identity, to release time from the human functions of narrative, we can turn to poetry. Because poetry tends to emphasize the associative nature of thought – focusing, for instance, on the centrality of metaphor to human experience rather than on narrative notions of plot – it can be especially well suited to investigating the slipperiness of consciousness. This opens some intriguing possibilities for poetry to experiment with representing sleep. Indeed, the poetry of sleep has often tended to double down on the non-narrative tendencies of poetic expression, venturing toward experimental ways of representing the dissolution of identity, coherence, and meaning. Whereas Proust's writing, by seeking to come closer and closer to the boundary that narrative can never cross, begins to challenge Reiss's proposal that it is "impossible to describe the condition of *being* asleep," poetry challenges this assertion in different terms, partly by questioning the assumption that description is the only way to represent experience.

For instance, experimental poet a. rawlings's long poem *Wide Slumber for Lepidopterists* rejects the conventions of narrative, description, and coherence. It presents the moth as a metaphor for sleep, yet this image is anything but straightforward. The use of the moth – a delicate, mysterious, fluttering nocturnal presence – as a figure for sleep is reasonably intuitive; indeed, television ads for Lunesta, a sleep drug manufactured by Sepracor, which coincidentally aired around the same time as the publication of *Wide Slumber for Lepidopterists*, famously featured an eerily glowing, animated green moth that fluttered from window to window as it alighted upon the backs of restless insomniacs, sending them into a deep, satisfying sleep.[9] rawlings's book explores the moth for entirely different reasons. A lepidopterist is a person who studies butterflies and moths, and rawlings's poetry draws a link between the clinical study of moths and the clinical study of sleep, such that the act of collecting the moth and pinning it for display inside a sealed box, which requires capturing and killing the specimen, implies that putting sleep on display for clinical study involves the contradictory notion of killing a living process in order to understand it. She develops this metaphor by splicing instructions for preserving the moth with often nonsensical streams of words meant to represent the experience of sleep:

> Inhale to sleep crows on crows of army worms; uncontrol cannibalistic owlet moths.
>
> *Relax dried specimen by placing in humid environment.*
>
> Welcome to the Centre for Sleep and Dream Studies. Welcme to th
>
> Enter. Sleep nd ream. elcm
>
> *Use fungicide to prevent mould growth on specimen.*
>
> nether leap, the flights, coalesceTHE#FLIGHTSimplode, coal[10]

Ironically, the insights into sleep that presumably should be provided by the Centre for Sleep and Dream Studies are rendered incoherent as the consciousness of the sleeping subject dissolves. The real truth about sleep, these lines suggest, takes shape through the lived experience of the sleeper, not through the supposedly objective gaze of the sleep lab and certainly not through the conventions of narrative. Representing this assertion through words on a page is thus a contradiction that requires breaking down both the meaning and the mechanics of written language as wakefulness fades into sleep.

Sure enough, later in the book rawlings expands the moth-as-sleep metaphor to reflect on textual representation, with the web of symbolism now including poem as moth and poem as sleep, suggesting that the act of representing and studying sleep on the page, even in an experimental book like this one, is just as precarious an endeavour as learning about the moth by killing it:

> specify comma, question mark? dissect comma? intersect question mark, comma?
>
> *Collect, sort and frame text.*
>
> *How does a text fall asleep?*
>
> *Pinch meaning between morpheme and phoneme.*
>
> *How does text eat itself?*
>
> *Slide meaning into envelope; store in box with semanticide.*[11]

Studying the experience of sleep through textual representation, much like pinching and pinning the corpse of the moth, requires the death of the living thing being examined. The collector (or the poet, or the reader) must be prepared to pin language down by placing it in a box (such as a book), where it is killed with "semanticide," a neologism referring to a substance that destroys meaning. That is to say, if capturing sleep in language destroys the lived experience of sleep, any poem about sleep has already destroyed itself. It only follows that a poetics of sleep would crumble into meaningless fragments. Yet, although killing the moth leaves the moth lifeless, killing the meaning in language may help the language to "fall asleep" in a more fruitful sense by embracing the dissolution of consciousness in the sleeper. The destruction of meaning within the poem paradoxically *creates* meaning by mirroring the experience of sleep.

Wide Slumber for Lepidopterists is difficult to understand, and that is part of the point, given the incomprehensibility of sleep. Many of the pages are truly nonsensical, not only at the level of words and phrases but also in the rejection of textual lineation, as broken words are often scattered across the page, refusing to indicate a coherent sequence of reading from left to right. The text, like the consciousness of the sleeper, becomes lost in a disordered chaos. Moreover, the sleep is not a peaceful sleep but is disrupted through an alarming number of sleep disorders, or parasomnias, that appear throughout the volume and that rawlings clarifies in a glossary; these include bruxism ("where the sleeper grinds or clenches her teeth"), circadian arrhythmia ("in which the sleeper does not adhere to a standard daily 24-hour pattern"), and sleep apnea ("repeated and temporary suspension of breath during sleep").[12] Interspersed among all of these disorders are images of sometimes passionate, sometimes violent sex – thrusting tongues, heavy breathing, pinned bodies, and penetration – which lead literary scholar Sarah Groeneveld to identify in the poem "a parallel between the lepidopterist who pins down moths and butterflies and the act of rape."[13] Groeneveld thus argues that although "the sleep cycle theme at first seems to be benign [it] quickly deteriorates into a nightmare."[14] This reading is especially meaningful given that the sexual assault of sleeping women by male partners is a much more pervasive societal problem than has usually been acknowledged.[15] Like an actual dream, *Wide Slumber* shifts between beauty and horror, from one vision to another, in ways that are difficult to resolve.

Does *Wide Slumber* perform an experiment with the dissolution of language – its own act of semanticide – in order to reflect as truthfully as possible the dissolution of consciousness during sleep? Or does the book use sleep as yet another metaphor in order to investigate the limitations of poetic expression, the illusion of scientific objectivity, and the forms of violence imposed on women and the environment? Groeneveld finds sleep to be only a secondary concern in the text; for her, *Wide Slumber* is primarily a comment on settler colonialism in Canada and is best illuminated by theories of ecocriticism and the postcolonial gothic, an assessment that may come as a surprise to some readers. The difficulty of developing a single or straightforward reading of the text speaks, among other things, to a key paradox in the representation of sleep within literature. A text that wants to examine the experience of sleep cannot easily rely on the conventions of narrative and language tied to waking life, which means that it immediately places its own status as a recognizable text under threat. Conversely, a text that illuminates sleep through clear language, elements of narrative sequence, or even the conventions of metaphor and symbolism may turn out to have little to say about sleep per se, using sleep merely as a vehicle for exploring other concerns. I look further at experimental sleep poetry, and what it might mean for a text to fall asleep, when I discuss Sandra Huber's *Assembling the Morrow* in chapter 4.

Part of the problem with the claim that we cannot describe the condition of being asleep is that it sees sleep as a singular event rather than a blended, layered set of shifting experiences. The fact, for instance, that one part of your brain might be a bit more asleep than another poses a major challenge to the view that sleep cannot be perceived. Another challenge emerges from hypnagogia, the transitional state from wakefulness to sleep characterized by hallucinatory half-dreams. Hypnagogia dispels the notion that the transition into sleep occurs in one instant. The passage into sleep is a gradual disordering of the landscape more than a single step through a dark doorway; it is a journey that conjures up strange creative opportunities. In the hypnagogic state, for instance, a person might experience a vision of "putting a horse into a sort of violin case and zipping it up" or other bizarre and creative formulations.[16] Intriguingly, then, hypnagogia and dreaming do not just allow for investigation in poetry but also actually take the form of wandering poetic experimentation, using imaginative expression to draw unexpected conceptual links.

Some of the most memorable works of sleep poetry explore these concerns, focusing less on experiments with the nature of textuality than on the arresting images and conceptual figures that might emerge during the hallucinatory passage into sleep. In his poem "Hypnagogia," Don Domanski writes,

> we travel through hypnagogia   not awake
> nor asleep   our minds all glitter
> and fingerpaint   our hearts turned to shadows
> our shadows re-envisioning the light of our true
> natures   while the ground of being rises and falls[17]

A mark of a good poetic image is that it causes us to see something familiar in a new way. The strange visions that occur on the boundary of sleep, figured beautifully here as the glitter and fingerpaint of the mind, can now be understood as the spontaneous artistry of a consciousness unconcerned with realism, or indeed with any expectations of representation. Glitter and fingerpaint are associated with the unaffected art of young children, the mind on the verge of sleep abandoning the adult notions of logic and planning in favour of visual wonder and magical thinking. The "ground of being" that "rises and falls" captures both the rhythmic expansion and contraction of the lungs as the resting body prepares for sleep and the shifting figurative ground of our sense of self, which fades, re-emerges, and fades again in hypnagogic vertigo. Shades of textual experimentation remain present here in the gaps between words and in the arresting moments of the sudden line breaks, as the use of language to represent sleep, like the sleeper's consciousness, rises, falls, and rises again.

Domanski's "Hypnagogia" might be taken as an example of how poetry can investigate sleep in two key ways: through experimental visions of the experience of sleep and through the development of theme through narrative. Many poems, after all, tell a story, and the interest in a given poem often emerges through the way that the telling of the story takes shape via formal elements such as repetition, variation, and line breaks. Looking at the thematic development of sleep within poetry is thus illuminating in its own right, and it forms a bridge to the examination of literary fiction, which I discuss in the next chapter.

Among the thematic concerns arising in sleep poetry is the unique role of sleep in human intimacy. The colloquial meaning of the phrase "sleeping with someone" to refer to sex may tend to overshadow the more literal meaning of the words, but sleeping alongside another sleeper is an intense figure for intimacy. We are, in a sense, never closer to another person than when we participate in the shared vulnerability and replenishment of sleep. Yet, because we lose ourselves in sleep, sleep also separates us from one another, paradoxically creating a profound disconnect within our closest moments. Poetry about sleep has found within this loss both a lamentation on and a window into the ambivalences of close relationships. In her 1981 poem "Variation on the Word *Sleep*," Margaret Atwood writes,

I would like to watch you sleeping,
which may not happen.
I would like to watch you,
sleeping. I would like to sleep
with you, to enter
your sleep as its smooth dark wave
slides over my head[18]

"I would like to watch you, / sleeping" is a near repetition of "I would like to watch you sleeping," but the comma and line break reverse the matter of who is doing the sleeping, an echo of the way that the shared experience of sleep brings about a disconnect. The obvious reading of this poem is that the speaker craves an intimacy so intense that it would involve entering her lover's sleep, that most personal and vulnerable realm. "I would like to sleep / with you" thus turns away from the metaphor of sleep as sex and instead introduces the more fantastic intimacy of inhabiting a shared sleep-world, as the speaker imagines the impossible act of joining her lover in his dreams. In the later stanzas of the poem, the speaker travels alongside the lover through the dangerous dreamscape, protecting him from his fears and eventually escorting him back to the waking world.[19]

Scholar Jill Hufnagel, however, develops a more intriguing reading of this poem; for Hufnagel, the speaker is "at once deeply enamored with the one she addresses and aggressively desirous of having power over him."[20] By virtue of becoming the lover's saviour, the speaker also becomes "a necessity for his preservation and, ultimately, for his existence," a menacing position that allows her "to compensate for the inabilities of her waking, passive persona."[21] In this reading, the speaker uses sleep as a vehicle for manipulation and power, as a site where she can live out the fantasy of making her lover fully dependent on her. And, indeed, the lover has no voice of his own in this poem; his existence is shaped entirely by the speaker's words. As Hufnagel points out, the speaker's description of the lover's dream – with its "wavering forest of bluegreen leaves" and its ominous cave of grief and fears – is a projection of the speaker's fantasies, not a description of what the sleeping lover might actually be seeing.[22] If shared sleep creates a paradox of intimacy and disconnection, Atwood's poem heightens the stakes of this contradiction, allowing itself to be read variously as a tender love poem and as a manifesto of power and control. Literary scholar Heather Heckman-McKenna similarly notes that "I would like to watch you sleeping" is a line that "might be perceived by different readers as intimate or voyeuristic or foreboding, and so on, dependent on the reader's associations with such an assertion."[23] By way of the "variation" in the poem's title, sleep is literal sleep, but it is also the centre of a solar system of symbolic associations, variously signifying intimacy, peacefulness, support, vulnerability, disconnection, threat, power, sex, trauma, and dreaming.

Leonard Cohen's 1964 poem "Two Went to Sleep" plays on a similar theme, as the poem's companion sleepers are perfectly synchronized in their shared act of sleeping yet embark on entirely separate, disconnected journeys through their individual dream lives:

> Two went to sleep
> almost every night
> one dreamed of mud
> one dreamed of Asia
> ...
> one bargained nicely
> one was a snowman
> one counted medicine
> one tasted pencils
> one was a child
> one was a traitor
> ...
> one night happy
> one night in terror
> Love could not bind them
> Fear could not either
> they went unconnected
> they never knew where[24]

The sleepers' experiences during the night are unpredictable and can never be shared. The two people are irremediably separate, yet they also share a companionship by virtue of undergoing the same mysterious experience at the same time. The poem does not distinguish the identities of the two sleepers but refers to both of them using the same word – "one" – paradoxically making each sleeper an isolated individual whose identity is shared with the other. Likewise, the lines "they went unconnected / they never knew where" show that even though the sleepers rove independently through their own slumber, "they" share a togetherness within this experience of solitary wandering. Sleep is an experience that is held in common even while it confirms the isolation of subjectivity.

Whereas "Two Went to Sleep" approaches sleep as a universal philosophical problem, poetry can also challenge generalizations about sleep in many productive ways, such as by recognizing the links between sleep and forms of inequity. In her volume *Thirsty*, Dionne Brand develops a vision of the agonies and complexities of life in the urban centre of Toronto:

> if it is late at night and quiet, as quiet
> as a city can get, as still as its murmurous genealogy
> you can hear someone's life falling apart
>
> Most people can sleep through a siren. I can't.
> It isn't the proximity of it that wakes me, as shores,
> it is its emotion. Its prophecy. Even at a great distance
> you sense its mortal discoveries[25]

These lines recall, but darken, the cliché about New York being the "city that never sleeps." Brand's city of Toronto indeed never becomes silent during the night, but she asserts that "most people" within the city routinely sleep through the noise, even though the sirens echoing through the streets signal "someone's life falling apart." That the city is quieter at night makes the trauma of the siren more pronounced, with the act of sleep being especially audacious. To sleep in such a place is to remain heedless of the pain unfolding all around, yet sleep is the choice that most people make; they "can" sleep through the sirens, so they do. The siren thus becomes a metaphor for the crises of strangers and sleep a metaphor for indifference. Sleep is central to Brand's vision of the city in both its figurative and literal forms, as her poetic speaker endures the struggle of actual sleepless nights brought about by her deep empathy. Another way of reading this scene would be to say that sleeping through the trauma of others is a necessary skill for survival in the city, a skill that Brand's speaker fails to acquire, making her a tragic outsider, a Cassandra figure whose endlessly open eyes must see what others do not see at the cost of her own sanity.

For Indigenous writers, sleep has taken form variously as a source of spiritual or cultural knowledge through dreams (which I discuss more in the next chapter in the context of novels), as a focal point for the painful disruptions of settler colonialism, and as a site of resistance or "survivance," this latter term emerging from the work of Anishinaabe scholar of Native American studies Gerald Vizenor. Survivance, he writes, is "an active sense of presence, the continuance of native stories, not a mere reaction, or a survivable name. Native survivance stories are renunciations of dominance, tragedy, and victimry."[26] Multiple visions of sleep, then, are important in their own ways. Indigenous poetry can present sleep as a figure that illuminates the traumas of residential schools and other embodiments of colonization or as a figure that asserts the existence of Indigenous forms of experience in their own right.

In his poem "Waking Up," Inuit writer Alootook Ipellie ironizes the colonial notion that traditional Indigenous societies, as though stuck in the past, are figuratively sleeping through the inevitable progress of modernity. Although the settler society might see itself as helping Inuit to "wake up" from the lethargy of their way of life, Ipellie sees this form of waking as a tragic and costly transformation:

> Waking up
> From what was literally
> A nomadic life the night before
> To a lifestyle where Inuit hunters
> Spend all their precious time
> Sitting in front of a computer
> Pushing predetermined buttons and keys
> That allow them to launch
> Rocket-powered harpoon missiles
> Arrows and fish-spears
>
> ...
>
> Waking up
> With a slap in the face

My preference is to go back to yesterday
And begin all over again

Tonight
I will think twice about going to sleep
I will be afraid of
Waking up[27]

The phrase "wake up" has been used as a call to action – as a protest against ignorance and complacency. Here, however, the phrase takes on a dark tone since the world into which the speaker has woken is, in effect, a nightmare. It is the Western technological society symbolized by computers, not the nomadic Inuit hunting culture, that involves an immobilized way of life, as the computer user sits inert (practically sleeping) at a terminal where all possible actions are mediated by a screen, prearranged by buttons, and tied to destructive automatic weapons. This troubled notion of waking up also casts the traditional Inuit way of life as a dream that evaporates in the harsh light of day, meaning that the desire to return to what has been lost ("My preference is to go back to yesterday") reflects an impossible nostalgia for a life that can never be restored. The final lines of the poem ("Tonight / I will think twice about going to sleep") suggest that the emotional weight of the loss of the hunting life is not a one-time disruption but a repeating experience of fear and dismay. Sleep, as a repetitive nightly event, is disrupted by anxiety on a literal level, even while it becomes a metaphor for recurring pain.

In Cree writer Rosanna Deerchild's poem "bread crumbs," the speaker is a child in the residential school system who, facing malnutrition, must stay awake at night to steal food:

after lights out
nuns and kids asleep
sneak out

one at a time
quick soundless
mice across floor

one props door
another steals bread
a third watches out

each night eat
only what we need
just enough to ease

stomach pain
crushing thirst
just enough to sleep[28]

In contrast to representations of the night as a time of comfort and security for children, this poem casts the sleeping hours as the only opportunity to fight the starvation imposed by the colonial "school." Significantly, the three children must keep their nighttime thievery secret not only from the nuns but also from the other children in the shared residence, who might be coerced into betrayal if they witness the theft. This need for secrecy sows the seeds of distrust among the children, turning what should be the peaceful hours of sleep into a time of suspicion and fear, creating a sense of urgency that is reflected in the sparse and halting phrasings in the poem. If they were caught, the children who sneak out of bed would be punished not only for the theft of food but also for not sleeping, yet the failure to sleep is caused by hunger in the first place. The children are ordered to sleep, which they cannot do until they steal food when they should be asleep – a cruel contradiction that, as in Ipellie's "Waking Up," turns sleep into a site of literal suffering as well as a figure for colonial brutality.

Another of Deerchild's poems, "mama making moccasins," creates a much more positive vision of sleep. Rather than being separated from her family, the speaker in this poem is in the company of her mother; the poem is a tender and attentive description of the mother's process of sewing a pair of moccasins, and it ends with the speaker falling asleep:

the night heavy with stars and beads
i fall asleep   to the sound
of humming and mama
making moccasins[29]

The figure of sleep here is precisely the opposite of the one in "bread crumbs," reflecting peace, replenishment, safety, and the continuity of the family. However, although reading these two poems in juxtaposition may be useful in order to contrast family togetherness with colonial damages, it is important to note that "mama making moccasins" does not frame itself primarily as a work of resistance or as a reaction to the residential schools. Rather, it develops a loving portrait of the Cree family, with the mother's thread, felt, and beads forming "her very own landscape."[30] As Vizenor's concept of survivance suggests, such a poem focuses not on victimhood or overcoming but on the continuance of Indigenous stories, brought to a coda here through an affirmation of the pleasures of sleep. Deerchild is not the only Indigenous poet to develop the figure of sleep in this way. A similar initiative takes shape, for example, in Ojibwe Anishinaabe writer Lesley Belleau's poem "Sunday at the Healing Lodge," where the speaker enters the lodge and says, "I glimpse the first recognition of mother / swallow the full peace in a newness of sleep. / my feet now connect to the ground."[31]

The problematic notion of sleep as a universal or neutral matter of personal experience can be challenged not only through attention to diverse cultural visions and matters of injustice but also through bodily experiences. In her poem "The Hot Women," Rhona McAdam portrays sleep loss in terms of menopause:

> Sleep spills from our beds. We rise
> in burning armies, hauled
> from the molten deep,
> to creak the halls, brittle
> and precarious
> on feet of fire.[32]

Contrary to the way that insomnia is so often understood as an individual problem – as something that a person can fix by practising the right mindfulness techniques or buying a new mattress – "The Hot Women" depicts sleep loss as an experience of suffering for menopausal women that is characterized by its being held in common. The use of the first-person plural ("our beds" and "we rise") alongside the imagery of fire and armies portrays the intense bodily heat of menopause as a force that is both dangerous and collective. Although the poem does not "solve" the problem of sleep loss, it does propose a form of solidarity and recognition, rejecting the notion that insomnia in middle-aged women is an individual neurosis or a failure that can be corrected through simplistic means.

Kelly Shepherd's poetry volume *Insomnia Bird: Edmonton Poems*, which won the Robert Kroetsch City of Edmonton Book Prize in 2019, considers the inequities of sleep within the urban environment. In the poem "Crescent," a woman is irritated about being woken by the landscaping crew that she has hired to spread rocks as ground cover beside her house: "If she had ordered sod to go there instead // of rock, she would still be sleeping."[33] Read on its own, this scene would appear entirely mundane. However, the poem opens with an epigraph from Indigenous rights scholar Peter Kulchyski:

> a person who relates to a building
> not as the site of meetings or a capital investment
> or a status symbol, but a warm air duct
> that promises the possibility of sleep,
> is living in the city as bush.[34]

Framed by this epigraph, the woman's irritation at being woken by her landscaping crew is embarrassingly trivial, as she is oblivious to the crisis of homelessness in the city. Just as the poem would be a fundamentally different poem without the epigraph, the ordinary business of one person's sleep reads differently when seen alongside someone else's, particularly in the context of poverty and colonization. The woman's decision to remake her small suburban plot of land becomes a microcosm of settler colonialism, and the disruption to her sleep hints at the uneasy repercussions of colonial land use, even while her sleep remains far more secure than the person who needs a warm air duct and whom she never meets. Context is everything, as the juxtaposition of these two experiences of sleep establishes a relationship between them, altering their identity and meaning.

In another *Insomnia Bird* poem, sardonically titled "Cultural Darwinism for Dummies," the speaker is a bookshop employee who, against the advice of his co-worker, gives the washroom key to a man with "grubby clothes // and unwashed hair."[35] The man doesn't return from the washroom, and eventually the speaker "opened the door // and there he was, stretched out asleep on the bathroom floor ... My co-worker had been right. / This was Edmonton in the winter time." The police are called, and later the speaker is embarrassed about having told the police the sleeping man's race, when he should have lied about it: "'He's Caucasian,' I should've said. / 'I think he's Asian,' I could've said." The poem doesn't specify the sleeper's race, although it implies that the speaker is anxious about reinforcing stereotypes about Indigenous people. As with "Crescent," the relatively comfortable position of members of the settler society – who control access to material necessities such as the washroom as well as the information and power symbolized by rows of expensive books – is disrupted by the presence of an impoverished person who is excluded from sleep within the urban environment. Here, too, the vexation experienced by the settler creates an opening – one that is given literal form in the moment when the speaker "opened the door" – through which the sleep of others can be reconsidered. The open doorway reveals the man asleep on the bathroom floor, thus making the speaker's frustration insignificant through its juxtaposition with extreme poverty.

In her poetic travelogue *Magnetic North: Sea Voyage to Svalbard*, Alberta poet Jenna Butler describes her experience as a writer in residence aboard a barquentine sailing ship in the Norwegian Arctic during a two-week voyage over the summer solstice.[36] Whereas much of her narrative focuses on the ravages of global heating visible in the receding glaciers, and on the communities of people on the islands of Svalbard whose lives are shaped by the extreme conditions of the Arctic Ocean, her descriptions repeatedly turn to the unsettling effects of the "long, bright nights."[37] "The sun," she writes, "is directly overhead twenty-four hours a day. Death leaps at me with the intensity of searchlights. Bones bleach and fissure over a matter of weeks."[38] The comment about the sun being directly overhead may be an exaggeration (the sun would actually be closer to the horizon), but the phrase accurately speaks to Butler's sense of inescapable misery, as there is no relief from the light. The endless glare leads immediately into images of death, as the ecosystem of the Arctic strikes Butler primarily as a collection of bleached bones crumbling in the harsh rays of constant sun. In the absence of the peace and replenishment of darkness, all that seem to remain are death and decay.

Indeed, Butler's poem called "Night" is actually about the lack of night, a problem that takes a fearful toll on the body. "There's no place to hide," she writes. "Night is non-existent, circadian cranked to overtime. No twilight, no dusk, no dawn ... Something in us paces, sleepless, sits on its haunches and observes morning rituals of black coffee."[39] The rote act of pouring a cup of coffee only emphasizes the fact that the notion of morning has lost much of its meaning. Although the people onboard the ship can physically lie down on their bunks, they never achieve a properly restful sleep but remain figuratively upright, squatting exhaustedly on their spiritual haunches. The destructive effects of the endless daylight (at least, through the eyes of an outsider who is new to the Arctic) thus migrate rapidly from the ecosystem into the sleepless soul of the individual witness.

Magnetic North could be read as a comment on how the grand notion of climate change, when seen up close, breaks apart into the intimacies of personal experience. What is particularly frightening about Butler's experience is that she cannot look away from the scenes of death and destruction that surround the ship, all of which gleam endlessly in "the intensity of searchlights." Trapped in constant daylight, she *must* bear witness. Like Brand's poetic speaker in *Thirsty*, she cannot help but see. "Darkness becomes mythic, vein-shot, red light through pinched eyelids," Butler writes. "What we took for granted: the relief of the dark. How concealment, too, is a sort of blessing ... We learn what the explorers knew: that darkness is not a right but an indulgence."[40] Because she can't look away from the illuminated world, she can't retreat from the glare of reality; there is no rest, no recovery, no way to block the light seeping in through closed eyelids. The relentless power of sight also means that there is no retreat from the gaze of others, no relief from scrutiny and responsibility. Sleeplessness, then, is the desperate absence of literal sleep, and it is also a metaphor for the inability to recover from what has been witnessed, the inability to withdraw from the harsh light of a deadly world.

Sleep, as an experience and a concept, is about much more than enhancing daytime productivity, and as these works reveal, poetry about sleep builds meaning through many different approaches, from experimental formal manipulation, to dreamlike imagery, to the representation of personal relationships. What is more, the concerns raised within many of these works, from the associative link between sleep and patriarchal violence, to the question of where impoverished people can sleep in a cold city, to the sleepless glare of the melting Arctic, indicate that sleep is frequently, and perhaps inevitably, tied to matters of politics, justice, and power. Building a critical awareness of sleep is about more than advocating for restful slumber or pushing back against the notion of sleep as a productivity enhancer; it must involve recognizing that the forms of comfort and security at stake within the realm of sleep extend far beyond concerns over blankets and pillows. When we talk about sleep, we rarely talk only about sleep, and poetry can bring to light the many shapes that sleep takes within language, culture, and imagination.

SLEEPLESSNESS IN *SLOW WAR*

Benjamin Hertwig's poetry volume *Slow War*, published in 2017, is a rich work that takes sleep as a key theme. Studying this text in detail shows how poetry can produce vital interventions into the conflict between competing cultural visions of sleep. When should sleep be seen as a site of cultural power tied to political concerns, and when should it be understood as a fraught bodily need? Or, just as importantly, how can we negotiate the frustrations and harms that emerge from the terms of this question? In *Slow War*, the battlefield for this dispute is the literal battlefield of military operations. The book challenges dominant representations of sleep in the context of war, especially by rejecting the notion that the peaceful figurative "sleep" of dead soldiers deserves its place of cultural honour as the definitive representation of sleep in war (a vision embodied in particular by John McCrae's poem "In Flanders Fields"). By presenting an insistent focus on the actual disruption of sleep for living soldiers and ex-soldiers, *Slow War* reclaims sleep from the figurative realm and brings it back to the literal. By challenging the dominant vision of sleep in war, it also challenges the cultural vision of war as a whole.

War is a particularly significant realm where sleep operates as a contested ground and where the physical need for sleep is placed under terrible stress. Observing that sleep deprivation poses a major problem for military operations, Simon J. Williams writes that "the commodification or customisation of sleep in medical, corporate or popular culture, is paralleled if not surpassed by its transformation into a commodity of war in the military; something to be managed, mobilised, modified."[41] Great amounts of funding have been committed to developing methods for tracking, manipulating, and perhaps someday eliminating the need for sleep among soldiers in order to create a strategic advantage.[42] Thomas Balkin, who studies behavioural biology for the US military, observes that "sleep has always been a weapon."[43] Alongside these intentional manipulations, however, sleep also becomes an unintended longer-term casualty of war, as sleep loss is a well-known problem for veterans. Indeed, the troubled sleep of veterans of the Vietnam War helped to establish the medical concept of post-traumatic stress disorder, and an American study in 2010 found that nearly two-thirds of veterans who served in Afghanistan and Iraq experience insomnia.[44]

It is unsurprising, then, that representations of sleep arise frequently in war literature, and that they serve diverse and contested functions. Visions of sleep in its symbolic association with death and a peaceful afterlife can be used to convince the population that the deaths of soldiers are proudly made sacrifices that serve a larger good, which in turn can bolster the war effort and persuade citizens to fight. In contrast, other representations of sleep can challenge the more heroic notions of war by reflecting not only how the realities of battle and military service can cause terrible sleep disruptions for those in the war but also how insomnia can tyrannize the lives of ex-soldiers. These latter visions tend to assert that the meaning of sleep should arise not from its figurative association with death but from its more literal existence as a biological need. Who can forget the scene in Timothy Findley's novel *The Wars* where "Robert had only taken eight hours' sleep in the last three days ... His body was completely numb and his mind had shrunk to a small, protective shell in which he hoarded the barest essentials of reason."[45] Robert is denied sleep as part of his involvement in the military order, and he loses his mind; the power of the imagery in this scene arises from intense physical agony, not from any romantic notion of sacrifice. Or, consider the speaker in Dionne Brand's poem *Inventory*, who cannot sleep because she is consumed by the need to keep track of the people killed by bombs, guns, and other forms of destruction: "a sleep, no, / sleep would be forgiving."[46] Sleep, for her, is certainly a physical necessity, yet because it cannot be disentangled from ethics and grief, it is also a form of meaning, a contradictory symbol of rest and anxiety.

Hertwig comes from a family with centuries-long military roots; his last name means "hard war."[47] After joining the Canadian Armed Forces at the age of sixteen, he was deployed to southern Afghanistan for six months in 2006. Among the events that he encountered during his tour of duty was a double suicide bombing of his convoy, which killed two Canadian soldiers. In an essay published eleven years after his return to Canada, he describes his political concerns regarding the conflicts in Iraq and Afghanistan, his unlikely friendship with former Al-Qaeda child soldier Omar Khadr after they met by chance in Edmonton, and, most powerfully, his ongoing experience of trauma as a former soldier. "When I first returned from Afghanistan," he writes, "the wrong question about my experience could derail my mind for days, putting me in a mental state from which I could not extricate myself."[48] The long shadow of this war has only become more apparent in the years since Hertwig's comments. In 2021, the US military withdrew from Afghanistan, resulting in a stunningly rapid takeover of the country by the Taliban. In addition to intensifying a humanitarian crisis for the people of Afghanistan, this event created a crisis of frustration and disillusionment for veterans of the war. Former Canadian reservist Bruce Moncur, who had to relearn how to walk, talk, and read after a severe battle injury in Kandahar, remarked that "we have been reduced to watching all our sacrifices wiped out in less than a fortnight."[49]

Slow War, which was a finalist for the Governor General's Literary Award in 2017, comprises over fifty poems that move back and forth, sometimes jarringly or confusingly, between the war zone in Afghanistan and civilian life in Canada. The formal approaches of the poems vary from finely structured sonnets and couplets to broken fragments of thought scattered across the page. The long afterlife of trauma is a primary concern in the poems, as the speaker's experiences and memories become caught up in the terrors of the war. Upon watching an Afghan soldier bleed to death, the speaker thinks to himself, "leave this city. / your short war is over."[50] That is to say, the long, slow war of post-traumatic stress has only just begun.

The matter of sleep arises in many of the poems in *Slow War*, usually hinting at a disturbing inversion of the nightly period of peace and recuperation and sometimes introducing a confusion between sleep and wakefulness that echoes the psychological confusion over being either in the war or not in the war, as in the lines "when you awake. / you are still / asleep, / waiting for war / to end."[51] In "Night Convoy, Kandahar," the "night" in the title of the poem is not a time of restfulness but a time of perilous travel along dark streets. Here, the "blanket weight / of protective plates / on your chest" is likened to the way "a mother / puts you to sleep."[52] The heaviness of the soldier's armour becomes a security blanket but a darkly ironic one given the intense danger. "Sleep" therefore also becomes ominous. What kind of sleep, exactly, would be induced by a blanket of battle armour? The notion of being "put to sleep" is particularly treacherous given the need for vigilance as well as the hint of death within the phrasing, and therefore the mother's role, too, becomes ambivalent. In the theatre of war, the infrastructure, sociality, and temporal patterns of sleep are turned upside down; what would normally be comforting is made hazardous.

The poem "Rumours, Forward Operating Base Wilson" describes violent reports of events from battle: Taliban forces torture captured soldiers; a sniper "stalks the hills in devil's flesh and devours men at a distance."[53] The speaker holds onto these reports not so much for their literal or strategic value but for a different reason: "they are just stories. and stories are for the slow hours at night when memory coagulates and you need to stay awake, or for noon when the sun is brightest and you need to fall asleep. stories are for pain. you wish to understand."[54] The ambivalence of the phrase "stories are for pain" leaves open the question of whether stories, like aspirin, are meant to counteract pain or whether they are useful because they accentuate pain, allowing nighttime wakefulness. Stories for pain keep the soldier awake at night and grant him sleep during the day, a function that he recognizes and values since he has internalized the need to subvert his own daily circadian experience. As the war defines his reality, he must learn how to undermine and rediscipline his own bodily patterns of sleep.

In "Somewhere in Helmand," the soldier's face is torn open: "face bleeding / flap of skin / size of a communion wafer."[55] These opening lines introduce the poem's disavowal of Christian salvation, as the transfigured blood and flesh of Holy Communion – the wine and the wafer of bread – become the actual blood and flesh of the injured soldier. He picks up his Bible and lies down behind the tire of a truck:

> head against the sand
> eyes on the book of
> genesis
>   fall asleep.
>
> ...
>
> wake to sand between
> silk white pages,
>   nothing much to say.[56]

Sleep here brings about a political awakening in which the redemptive power of religion is rejected. The Book of Genesis, which contains the narrative of creation and humanity's awakening into consciousness, causes the soldier to fall asleep, and the newly woken soldier then realizes that the Bible is an empty text containing nothing of value. The line "nothing much to say" applies not only to the Bible but also to the soldier, and indeed to the poet, since these words end the poem. The process of sleep and waking has eliminated Christianity as the word of authority, yet it has not offered up any replacement for what has been lost. The soldier's act of falling asleep and then waking up echoes the death and resurrection of Christ, furthering the link between the two that is established in the opening lines about the blood and the wafer. However, the soldier's awakening to blank pages – mere sheets of paper that are no longer described as a Bible, as Genesis, or even as a book – ironizes the notion of the actual Christ figure, who has disappeared entirely. One of the purposes of sleep is to consolidate knowledge, to build a sense of coherence out of the chaotic memories and impressions of waking life, but in the case of the soldier at war, the consolidation of knowledge means the disavowal of any higher authority or salvation. To wake from sleep is to open one's eyes only to cold irony.

The most notable encounter with sleep in *Slow War* occurs in "Somewhere in Flanders / Afghanistan," a poem that bitterly responds to Canada's most famous war poem, John McCrae's "In Flanders Fields." McCrae's poem, written in 1915 when he was a surgeon in the Canadian Field Artillery during the First World War, has been used to bolster support for the military and to recruit new soldiers.[57] Its most visible function, as a recitation each Remembrance Day in Canada, has been to rehearse, and thus to shape, the collective public memory regarding the sacrifice and heroism of war. The poem has been the central document in shaping this cultural vision in Canada for more than a century.

Although the gentle poppy is the most famous image in McCrae's poem, the final stanza troubles the peaceful swaying of the flowers in the breeze. The voices of the dead soldiers end the poem with a distinct warning, an explicitly sleep-related threat:

> Take up our quarrel with the foe
> To you, from failing hands, we throw

The torch: be yours to hold it high
If ye break faith with us who die,
We shall not sleep, though poppies grow
In Flanders fields[58]

The ghostly soldiers who have sacrificed their lives for the war effort now threaten guilt over their own sleeplessness as the punishment for any members of the living who might neglect to continue the battle against "the foe." As literary scholar Cynthia Sugars observes about the poem's ghostly speakers, because "our fallen comrades, our national heroes and compatriots, threaten us with a curse," the poem "emblematizes Canadians' own conflicted relation to their ancestral dead."[59] Indeed, the threat of ancestral insomnia may be difficult to evade given that the terms of the quarrel are unclear. Scholars such as Nancy Holmes and Mark McCutcheon have observed that since the foe is unnamed, it can stand in for any enemy, meaning that the nation can mobilize the poem in the service of any future war effort whatsoever.[60] Sleep here serves in its habitual figurative role as a metaphor for the peaceful "rest" of a dead body and for the remembered spirit of the person who once lived. In the poem's vision of society's obligation to continue the war effort, this figurative sleep hangs in the balance, as the insomnia of the dead soldiers threatens to haunt the living.

Both Holmes and McCutcheon also comment on the poem's reference to opium; the soldiers are so upset at the thought of betrayal that they cannot rest peacefully, even though they lie underneath a crop of poppies, whose extract, as McCutcheon says, induces "pharmaceutical sleep and forgetting."[61] In their insomnia, the dead cannot be released from the burden of remembrance that should rightfully belong to the living. To allow them to sleep, we must be the ones who remember. The conventional notion of the sleeping soldier as a figure that conjures respectful remembrance seemingly grants the dead permission to release themselves from the concerns of the world, but this release is always potentially withheld because the public's behaviour might be inadequate. In Canada's war imagery – which includes more literal images such as the 1918 victory bonds poster shown here – sleep is a form of manipulation, a psychological instrument meant to compel the citizenry to act in accordance with the desires of the nation-state.

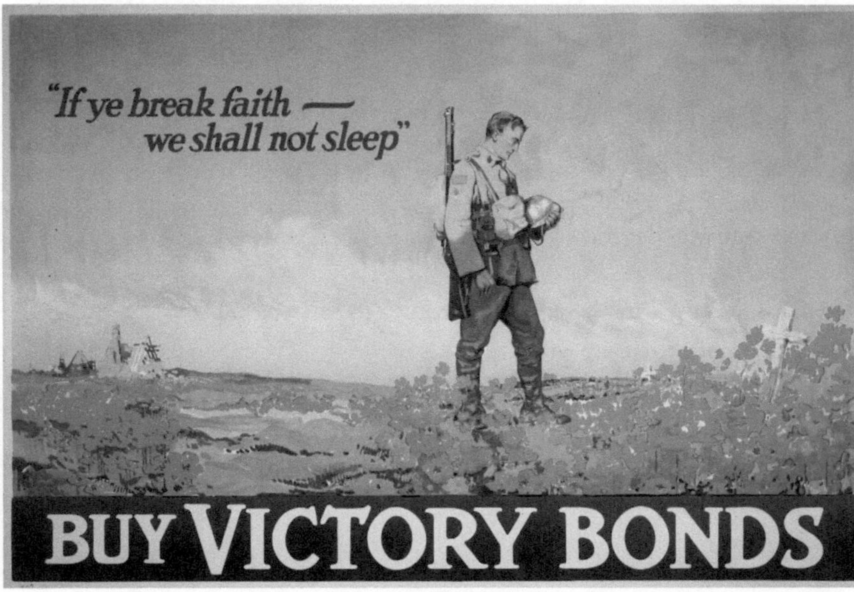
"If ye break faith —
we shall not sleep"
BUY VICTORY BONDS

2.1 "Buy Victory Bonds," campaign poster, 1918.

Hertwig's poem "Somewhere in Flanders / Afghanistan" challenges McCrae's representation of war, focusing ultimately on the strategic use of the figure of sleep:

> in Flanders Fields some shit
>   went down –
>
> flowers, crosses, the dead, etc. etc.
> but the dead do not speak John.
> ...
> *carthago delenda est*, so on so forth.
> you served our country, whatever
> that means.
>
> but I'm tired of hearing you go on
> about birds and sunsets and torches
> and god knows what else.

I'd rather meet your hundred-year-old
ghost on remembrance day.
when everyone's drinking to forget

the shit we volunteered to do
in a country that wasn't our own.

I'll buy you a beer though I don't really
drink much since my wife left,

don't sleep much either.

nobody sleeps well after
war.[62]

The use of "somewhere" and the interchangeability of Flanders and Afghanistan in the poem's title pick up on the unspecified nature of the foe, emphasizing the way that McCrae's poem allows for an uneasy blending of whichever enemies or theatres of war might emerge at any given moment. All wars, in a sense, become one long, protracted, slow war.

The bitterness and anger toward McCrae's, and thus the nation's, vision of war is not subtle but evident in the erasure of the poppies behind "some shit," the dismissal of McCrae's tedious concerns with "etc. etc.," and the insolent use of the colloquialism "whatever" left hanging before the line break. The line "*carthago delenda est*" ("Carthage must be destroyed") is a warmongering phrase of rhetorical fame used during the Roman Republic and deployed in the cause of all manner of geopolitical conflicts for more than two thousand years. In a commentary on Hertwig's poem, literary scholar Jonathan McGregor notes that the Latin phrase is "an invitation to the endless grudge match of history" and that, for Hertwig, "it is this imperative itself that must be destroyed."[63]

Sleep can be said to arise in the poem when Hertwig's speaker, who is "tired," imagines buying a beer for McCrae's "hundred-year-old / ghost," a meeting that would prevent McCrae's spirit from sleeping, as it were, in eternal peace. This envisioned meeting would occur on Remembrance Day, when for McCrae, the dead soldiers beneath their poppies should be released into sleep and forgetting, whereas for Hertwig, the living veterans are "drinking to forget" – a futile task, as the word "forget" leads inevitably into a recollection of "the shit we volunteered to do." The meeting with McCrae ironizes the threatened insomnia from "In Flanders Fields" by *ensuring* that the dead soldier is kept awake alongside the living one. McCrae must now bear witness to the insomnia of those who remain alive, just as Hertwig's speaker, who has survived his deployment in Afghanistan, suffers from trauma-related problems signified by alcohol and the separation from his wife, culminating in the loss of much of his ability to sleep.

We may wish to read this vision of McCrae as a personification of his famous poem rather than as a comment on the actual historical figure; after all, McCrae spent more time as a pathologist than as a soldier and war poet. Although Hertwig's poem chastens McCrae, it more importantly shames the cultural vision of war and remembrance for the belief that the sleep of the dead alone must be protected, when in fact the living soldiers and living ex-soldiers are paying the price of war with their insomnia. In doing so, the poem reclaims the notion of sleep, resurrecting it, as it were, from the ghostly realm of the figurative and returning it to the very present realm of the literal. The final lines of the poem – "nobody sleeps well after / war" – hint at a more conciliatory tone, as Hertwig acknowledges that he and McCrae share the common experience of insomnia. The enjambment that requires us to linger on the word "after" may call to mind the afterlife that McCrae so restlessly occupies. McCrae is denied his figurative sleep after life, and Hertwig is denied his literal sleep after war. The anger and the insistence on literal sleep remain present in these final thoughts, even while the closing line recognizes war to be the common enemy.

In the context of critical sleep studies, *Slow War* certainly belongs to what Williams calls the critical-reflexive agenda. This agenda is visible, for instance, in the way that the poems develop a sense of how the large-scale manipulation of sleep in the military can be internalized by individual soldiers, who must pay a price in terms of circadian normalcy, psychological stability, and conceptual orientation toward sleep. However, the question of a sleep-positive agenda is more complex. For Williams, a sleep-positive approach is one in which sleep is "championed ... through a variety of sleep-positive, sleep-promoting or sleep-friendly ideas and ideologies."[64] It would be reductive to say that *Slow War* simply advocates for good sleep. Rather, one of the key interventions of the text is that it identifies a conceptual battleground between different notions of what sleep means. The poems participate in, and challenge, the dangerous dance between the literal and figurative orientations toward sleep that circulate within the national collective consciousness. Whereas some of the poems insist on recognizing sleep and sleep loss as very literal problems, others advance pointed figurative meanings for sleep that emphasize danger, trauma, or disillusionment. In the case of "Somewhere in Flanders / Afghanistan," we might even say that the poem wants to destroy sleep, in the sense of the romanticized vision of dead soldiers. Sleep in these poems is both a physical need and a contested ground where power is negotiated, both a bodily experience and a site of intense cultural politics, both reality and representation. The poems develop a literacy of sleep in its physical, cultural, and representational contexts, honing a sense of when sleep should be protected and when it should be broken down.

3

Fictions of Sleep

SLEEP MAY BE ONE of the mundanities that usually seems to be absent from works of fiction, yet the representation of sleep in novels and other narratives has a surprisingly rich history. When sleep and sleeplessness appear in narrative fiction, they tend to operate in the service of a particular thematic interest, often to do with forms of inequity, trauma, or frustration. The sleep of characters who do manage to achieve restful slumber may indicate healing, acceptance, intimacy, or growth, and the implications of these elements reflect diverse contexts and concerns. As Michael Greaney asserts in *Sleep and the Novel*, "one way in which we invent sleep ... is by writing about it."[1] His investigation tends to illuminate how novels approach the comparative value of sleep and wakefulness, yet as his open-ended comment about inventing sleep implies, works of literature can produce meaning through sleep in a great many ways. In Canada, the dreams and slumbers of characters in fiction circulate within a particular set of social values, expectations, and histories. Whereas "In Flanders Fields" concerns itself with grand ideas about the nation, most literary representations of sleep in Canada develop more nuanced approaches, exploring how the meanings of sleep, as well as its material conditions, are shaped within specific contexts. Taken together, such visions of sleep identify the aesthetic possibilities of the literary imagination, and they also illuminate the nature of the cultural world – with all its possibilities and hazards – from which such an imagination might spring.

When it comes to understanding the representation of sleep in fiction emerging from Canada, especially as it relates to matters of culture, justice, and power, works by Indigenous writers require particular attention. As with the works of Indigenous poetry discussed in the previous chapter, Indigenous novels approach sleep from diverse points of view, often with an emphasis on the imperative of survivance as a way to assert the renewal and continuation of Indigenous cultures. Many works also confront the legacies of harm brought about by settler colonialism in Canada. In Lee Maracle's novel *Daughters Are Forever*, for example, the colonizers arrive on Turtle Island and carry out a vicious campaign of murder and destruction, but one woman who survives the attack finds the ability to recover through a combination of Westwind's advice and repeated sleep.[2] For Lisa, the Haisla protagonist of Eden Robinson's *Monkey Beach*, searching for her lost brother requires a method of contacting the dead. "Sleep is an altered state of consciousness," she learns. "To contact the spirit world, you must control the way you enter this state of being that is somewhere between waking and sleeping."[3] Sleep and sleeplessness can function variously as signals of colonization and as complex and positive assertions of cultural identity.

Jonny Appleseed is the first novel by Joshua Whitehead, an Oji-Cree member of Peguis First Nation on Treaty 1 land in Manitoba. The book won the 2019 Lambda Literary Award for gay fiction, and in 2021 it became the first book by an Indigenous writer to win CBC's Canada Reads. Whitehead identifies as Two-Spirit, and much of his writing addresses the need to assert and embrace Two-Spirit existence, both within Indigenous communities, whose internal recognition of gender roles has been affected by colonization, and within settler societies. Settler gender classifications, such as "transgender," although legitimate in their own right, don't correspond to the Indigenous term "Two-Spirit," which refers to "a person who identifies as having both a masculine and a feminine spirit."[4] Jonny, the protagonist of *Jonny Appleseed*, is a Two-Spirit Oji-Cree member of Peguis First Nation who moves to Winnipeg, where he earns an income running personal-webcam cybersex appointments for clients. In addition to the traumas of poverty and colonization, Jonny faces intolerance toward Two-Spirit people both on and off the reserve. Much of the narrative focuses on Jonny's efforts to navigate these conditions while he prepares to return to Peguis for the funeral of his stepfather.

The matter of sleep arises in the novel as a form of intimacy and healing, largely through Jonny's treasured relationship with his *kokum* (Cree for "grandmother"). After his kokum's death, Jonny recalls, "I stayed in bed and slept all day, every day ... My kokum had always told me that sleep was not a waste of time, that it was a time for healing, so I slept long and hard, waiting for my blood to leech out its memories and for my body to rejuvenate."[5] In a narrative that portrays the effects of multiple forms of trauma caused by colonization, poverty, and gender discrimination, the property of healing grants sleep a special significance. Moreover, that Jonny learns about the importance of sleep from his kokum emphasizes the intergenerational links that enable the continuity of cultural knowledge.

Sure enough, the many instances of good sleep in the novel are tied to forms of intimacy that foster replenishment and hope. Characters often fall asleep nestled into a loved one's body or lying tenderly on their lap. Jonny notes that "my head is the most sensual area on my body. When someone runs their hands through my hair and gently applies pressure on my temples, I can fall asleep on a dime. My mom and kokum used to put me to sleep this way when I was a kid."[6] Kokum in particular is very accepting of Jonny's gender expression, and he recalls that "she would apply her powders and lotions to my face with such grace and softness that I would fall asleep, smelling of talc and lilac."[7] He notes that his "favourite feeling in the world was when she clawed my hair with her fingers to put me to sleep" – a gesture that he desperately tries to recreate while nestled alongside her in a hospital bed after she takes her last breaths.[8] Sleep, then, both expresses and brings about the conditions of acceptance, safety, and care within the family structure. Even though Jonny spends much of the novel describing the pleasures of cigarettes, food, and sexual encounters, his "favourite feeling in the world" is that of his kokum granting him the replenishment and security of good sleep.

In this context, the scenes throughout the novel where Jonny *fails* to sleep well become particularly significant, as sleeplessness represents not only physical suffering but also the pronounced absence of intimacy, safety, and care. Although the novel is mostly character-driven, a central plot-based challenge for Jonny is that he has only two days to earn enough money to pay for a ride back to Peguis to attend his stepfather's funeral. He rises to this challenge by trying to double or triple his usual number of clients, who pay, on average, "twenty dollars a pop for a webcam peek-a-boo, at roughly twenty minutes per session."[9] This arrangement means that Jonny must run "all-night webcam sessions," thus sacrificing his sleep to carry out a repetitious and exhausting performance of intimacy that is made artificial by the mediation of the computer screens as well as by the context of sex work.[10] Elsewhere in the story, Jonny's sleep takes the form of blackouts after a night of binge-drinking with friends, such that time, memory, and agency disappear beneath the dangers of booze-fuelled unconsciousness, leaving Jonny unsure what has happened when he wakes up the next day.[11] "We used depressants," he says, "to offset our deep depression."[12] Blackouts may share with sleep a suspension of consciousness, but they are a perversion of the good sleep that kokum links with healing. Indeed, Jonny's failure to sleep alongside his kokum's body in the hospital, when he rests her hand across his head to mimic her old soothing gesture, indicates that he will have a hard time finding good sleep and rejuvenation without the familial support that she represents, as his troubled relationship with sleep becomes tied to the false comfort of alcohol and to the endless performance of intimacy for strangers.

Although criticism on *Jonny Appleseed* has tended to focus on the representation of Two-Spirit identity and on what literary scholar Lydia R. Cooper calls "queer digital sovereignty" in reference to how online communications are used in the story,[13] one might also say that the novel can be understood as Jonny's struggle to find good sleep since he must learn to reinforce the link between sleep and care while overcoming the damaging forms of sleep and sleeplessness that are tied to trauma, intolerance, and poverty. Significantly, in one of the novel's final scenes, when Jonny's lover, Tias, is distraught over the memory of his young sister, who was taken away by the foster care system, Jonny reproduces the gesture toward sleep taught to him by his kokum: "I pulled him back into the bed, lay his head in my lap ... I pricked my fingers as they grazed the sides of his head where his hair was buzzed, then ran them over to the top where his hair clumped together in dirty curls ... but he had fallen asleep by then."[14] Even though Jonny's own sleep remains deeply imperfect, he has learned to grant good sleep to his loved one, embodying the continuation of intimacy and familial protection that his Elders have passed down as an intergenerational imperative.

Literary texts are frequently populated by sleepers who fail to sleep, and contrary to the notion that sleeplessness is mainly a matter of poor sleep hygiene or lumpy pillows, this motif often involves links to discrimination in terms of gender and race. Even works that may not overtly take sleep as a central concern can illuminate these links, particularly in cases where the author speaks from within a marginalized group. Indeed, sometimes an understated appearance of sleep or sleeplessness within a text that is largely concerned with the effects of racism can suddenly expand the meaning of sleep loss, portraying it as an often hidden consequence of systemic discrimination.

For an example of the depiction of the politics of race that will be familiar to many students, we might turn to Rohinton Mistry's much anthologized 1987 short story "Squatter," which condemns Canada's late-twentieth-century notion of multiculturalism for its refusal to recognize the protagonist, Sarosh, an immigrant from India, as a "real" Canadian. The story is rarely, if ever, read as having anything to say about sleep, yet perhaps the most haunting image at the climax of the story is a depiction of the effects of sleep loss on the racialized protagonist. After failing for ten years to use a toilet in the Canadian way with a seated posture rather than a squat, Sarosh has given up on being Canadian and has boarded a plane from Toronto back to Bombay. However, in the airplane washroom, just before takeoff, he finally succeeds in his defecatory endeavour. Panicked, he tells a flight attendant that he must get off the plane even though it is already on the runway. "The wild look in his sleepless eyes, and the dark rings around them scared her," Mistry writes. "She beckoned for help."[15] The dehumanizing effects of marginalization have prevented Sarosh from sleeping, and this insomnia in turn only amplifies his grotesqueness, turning him into a "wild" creature who frightens the flight attendant into calling for reinforcements to secure him in his seat. Much of the writing in "Squatter" is satirical and humorous, yet Sarosh's sleep loss presents a disturbing image; his sleeplessness is both a symptom of a hypocritical model of multiculturalism that forces immigrants to change their most intimate habits and an emblem of his outsider status, a stain that marks him as a threat to the social order.

Far from being an isolated instance, the image of racialized sleep loss resonates painfully throughout Canada's longer history of exclusionary racist practices. In his novel *All That Matters*, Chinese Canadian writer Wayson Choy describes intense poverty among unemployed Chinese labourers in Vancouver in the 1930s. During their seasonal jobs, the men live in "a shift-time room, often just a bed with three or four others taking their turn to sleep; dozens had already starved to death, their bodies found in the rooming houses."[16] Once the jobs disappear, even the shared rooms are unaffordable, and the men take refuge in shacks and lean-tos on the outskirts of Chinatown. Some of the other Chinatown residents offer their warehouses and basements as shelters, where the homeless guests can be heard coughing up blood during the night.[17] Racist policies have banned Chinese people from becoming citizens or working in professions, thus creating inhumane, even deadly, conditions marked by torturous sleep.

David Chariandy's novel *Brother* takes up a contemporary consideration of systemic racism and immigrant life in Canada. The narrator, Michael, and his brother, Francis, who are the children of Trinidadian immigrants, live with their mother in Scarborough, an area of Toronto known for its cultural diversity and immigrant populations. The theme of confinement, of being trapped within their family history and within a social position characterized by poverty and violence, shapes much of the narrative. Michael's home, for example, is both sanctuary and prison, a place where he can take refuge from the pressures and exhaustion of the outside world but where he also finds himself trapped in impoverishment and grief. It is within this context that sleep arises as a painful absence tied to systemic poverty for Black immigrants. Michael's mother works lengthy shifts in cleaning jobs throughout the sprawling city, and she is always on the lookout for extra work that might help to fulfill "her vision of eventual arrival," even though the long hours mean "leaving her two young boys alone at home."[18] Michael notes that "if she learned the evening before of an impending night shift, she would spend precious sleep time cooking and worrying over the details of meals and activities for the following day."[19] As a member of the working poor, she must sacrifice one night of sleep in order to further sacrifice her sleep on the following night, all while feeling that she is never present enough for her kids.

Even for the neighbours who manage to sleep at night, sleep is not a refuge from their troubles but a precarious, vulnerable position that can be shattered at any moment. After Michael and Francis witness the shooting death of a drug dealer acquaintance on the street, the police arrive and capture the two brothers. Then, deciding that Michael and Francis had not been involved in the shooting, the police take the brothers home to their doorstep, where they tell the boys' exhausted mother that "a stray bullet had pierced the thin wall of a unit and struck a sleeping seven-year-old girl."[20] The tragedy of the girl being shot is heightened by the fact that she was in the sanctuary of her bedroom, engaged in an act that should represent innocence, safety, replenishment, and respite from the troubles of poverty and violence. If there is no safety in the sleep of a child, there is no safety anywhere. Meanwhile, the neighbours have been woken from their own slumber, drawn to stand in doorways watching the police talk to Michael's mother while the arriving news media vans flood the decaying apartment buildings with harsh television lights, turning the people's homes into a spectacle of poverty and crime – "our neighbourhood," Michael says, "now a crime scene cast hard in the clashing brightness of emergency."[21] In this way, the novel intensifies the theme of entrapment by showing that even sleep offers no escape, a notion that is further developed by the characters' sleeping arrangements throughout the rest of the story – in bedrooms shared with multiple siblings, among milk crates in the back room of a barbershop – which often serve as reminders of their poverty.

Moreover, several times throughout the novel, Michael's family members relive trauma as they make the transition into sleep. Chariandy repeatedly uses the phrase "the edge of sleep" in these moments, positing an image that brings to mind a precipice or, perhaps, the blade of a knife that penetrates the mind. Michael notes of Francis that "he'd be on the edge of sleep when some terror would visit him. He'd wake screaming a deep body scream, all cracked throat and emptied stomach, and it would take me a while to realize that I'd been screaming too."[22] After Francis is killed, their mother, in a desperate confusion at night, tries to reach him on the phone. "I knew," Michael says, "that only for a moment, on the edge of sleep, my mother imagined there was a country code she could dial, a toll she could pay."[23] Shortly after this, Michael repeats the phrase for a third time, now in reference to himself: "And now, on the edge of sleep, the shootings return to me with an attack of panic and wild vertigo."[24] Through these events and repetitions, the narrative links sleep conceptually with violence and trauma, tearing apart the more conventional link between sleep and peace. (We might recall Don Domanski's rendering of hypnagogia as the glitter and fingerpaint of the mind, an image whose sense of magic and wonder has no place in Michael's Scarborough.) Sleep deprivation becomes a spiral of cause and effect, even contributing to the most traumatic event in the novel. As an exhausted Francis realizes that the success promised by a deejay audition for a big record label had been a lie, Michael notices that "it all seemed to suddenly catch up with my brother: the sleepless nights after the shootings and before the audition."[25] Francis reaches a breaking point and attacks the venue's bouncers, suffering a severe beating and descending into reckless anger before being shot and killed by the police.

Yet, despite the intense pain associated with sleep, the characters in *Brother* cannot avoid the human need for slumber, and they must return to it each night as best they can. In doing so, they reinforce what literary scholar Paul Barrett sees as a central initiative in the novel: to recognize "how one might live with grief without forever living in its shadow."[26] For some readers, the representation of sleep in this story may serve as a validation of lived experience, whereas for readers who would not normally encounter the notion of sleep in the way that these characters do, what sleep *means* is changed by the novel in a way that requires sensitivity to the inequities tied to racialization and systemic poverty.

Michael Ondaatje's novel *The English Patient* develops a notable and problematic relationship between sleep and gender, illuminating how sleep can function in both literal and symbolic terms in the context of the patriarchal denial of female agency. One of the main female characters in the novel is Katharine, described to the reader through the recollections of the English patient (a mysterious figure generally referred to as Almásy). Katharine is a strong and memorable character in certain ways, yet she is heavily sexualized, taking form primarily through her passionate, adulterous affair with Almásy. In one of the novel's most memorable scenes – made especially famous by the 1996 film adaptation – a plane crash deep in the desert near the Egyptian-Libyan border leaves Katharine mortally injured and alone with Almásy, now her ex-lover. Taking her into a cave, he wraps her in a parachute for warmth and explains to her that he is going out to find help. Unable to return for three agonizing years, Almásy finally makes his way back to the cave to retrieve her body:

> She was still there. She had dragged herself into a corner, had wrapped herself tight in the parachute material ... She was on her back, positioned the way the mediaeval dead lie.
>
> I approached her naked as I would have done in our South Cairo room, wanting to undress her, still wanting to love her ... I lifted her into my arms from the shelf of sleep. Clothing like cobweb. I disturbed all that.[27]

This language, especially the line "I disturbed all that," creates a strange ambiguity about whether he has sex with her body. At the very least, he approaches her as a lover and trespasses physically upon her sleeping form. In other words, Katharine is a Sleeping Beauty figure and Almásy is the prince.

Cressida Heyes notes that the "Sleeping Beauty" fairy tale reflects a particularly assertive patriarchal vision of gender roles. Upon entering puberty, Little Briar Rose falls into an enchanted sleep, which "signals a period of the ultimate passivity, in which the suspended animation of the young woman provides a backdrop against which history progresses – a history driven by men."[28] Sleep, then, becomes a metaphor for the absence of female agency in a world dominated by male action, a trope that finds its climax in the prince's act of kissing the young woman who is not conscious or able to consent. This sexual act awakens Little Briar Rose, whose life can proceed only when she has been chosen as a wife.

Almásy's lifting of Katharine's body also closely echoes an earlier story, "Sun, Moon, and Talia," collected in *The Pentamerone*, a fifteenth-century volume by Italian fairy tale collector Giambattista Basile. This version features a king who stumbles upon a lord's daughter, Talia, during her enchanted sleep. Upon seeing Talia's sleeping form, the king "felt his blood course hotly through his veins in contemplation of so many charms; and he lifted her in his arms, and carried her to a bed, whereupon he gathered the first fruits of love"[29] – that is to say, he rapes her, impregnating her with twins. Talia later wakes up, immediately assumes the role of loving mother, and goes on to marry the king, despite not having been conscious during the conception or the pregnancy. Although she is ostensibly the protagonist of the story, Talia has little agency even when she is awake.

Much as "Sleeping Beauty" has been reshaped through multiple tellings, Almásy relates the story of the plane crash and Katharine's waiting in the cave more than once. In one telling of the scene, Katharine whispers a few words of reproach about their affair, asking Almásy, "How did you hate me?" In another telling, she does not speak at all while Almásy ruminates on her beauty.[30] Katharine's voice and agency, so visible in other sections of the novel, are thus gradually reduced until she enters her timeless slumber, where she spends years waiting for the male protagonist to move the plot forward by touching her body, lifting her up figuratively from "the shelf of sleep." Whereas Little Briar Rose and Talia both wake up and fulfill their feminine childbearing duties, Katharine, whose sleep is actually death, cannot achieve even this constrained form of awakening, making her fairy tale both more tragic than the traditional stories and in a sense more committed to male agency.

The other main female character in the novel is Hana, a nurse who tends to Almásy, her mysterious wounded patient, around the clock. "At night he is never tired enough to sleep," Ondaatje writes. "She reads to him from whatever book she is able to find … Sometimes at two a.m. he is not yet asleep, his eyes open in the darkness."[31] In the ruined Italian villa where the patient rests in bed, Hana "preferred to be nomadic in the house with her pallet or hammock, sleeping sometimes in the English patient's room, sometimes in the hall, depending on temperature or wind or light."[32] She spends much of the novel this way, at one point telling her lover, Kip, "I am so tired, Kip, I want to sleep … I just want to close my eyes without thinking of others, want to find the crook of a tree and climb into it and sleep."[33] As Almásy gradually recounts the story of his time in the desert with Katharine, it becomes clear that one of Hana's main functions in the novel is to sacrifice her own sleep to care for a man so that he can explain his version of events at length.

Both of the main female characters in *The English Patient* are thus defined by their relationship to sleep but neither of them by the actual act of restful sleeping. One sacrifices her literal sleep to care for a man, and the other enters a figurative sleep in order to wait for a man to act. Commenting on the novel's attempt to reproduce the "Arthurian grail" romance genre, literary scholar Bill Fledderus observes that "Hana and Katharine are in many ways adjuncts to a symbolically more important male … At its most basic level Ondaatje's female character palette seems limited to either madonna or whore, nurturing saint or temptress."[34] Arthurian motifs notwithstanding, Ondaatje is a remarkably nuanced writer, and it may be reductive to see the gendered representation of sleep in this novel as a simple patriarchal trope. For instance, one might say that Katharine's inability to wake up after being touched by the male protagonist is a comment on the impossibility of feminine agency under a relentless, self-obsessed patriarchy. Such a scene may lead us to reflect that Little Briar Rose and Talia, too, never really wake up if the only role that they are able to fulfill in waking life is a preprogrammed one initiated without their consent. Nevertheless, it is difficult not to notice the striking limitations of Ondaatje's female characters, a problem that comes about largely through a gendered vision of sleep in both its literal and figurative forms.[35]

Although insomnia in fiction often signals that a protagonist is in distress, trauma in some cases manifests as *excessive* sleep. For a despairing character, sleep embodies the paradox of grief; sleep is both an active decision to take charge of one's healing and a helpless renunciation of agency in the face of unbearable pain. In Angie Abdou's novel *The Bone Cage*, Sadie swims obsessively, her entire life revolving around the pool as she undertakes years of training in preparation for the Olympics. However, when her grandmother dies, Sadie crawls into bed, her athletic regime coming to a crashing halt. "Sadie releases herself into that first deep, dark hole of sleep," Abdou writes, "and decides not to come out. She misses her first morning practice in a decade, sleeps dreamlessly straight through it."[36] Sadie spends three full days in bed, as though physically pulled under the blankets by the weight of her grief. In Cree-Métis writer Tracey Lindberg's novel *Birdie*, Bernice moves to British Columbia to try to escape a life of trauma, abuse, and precarity in Alberta. She lies down in bed and enters a dreamlike existence, a "sleepingwake state," which lasts for weeks.[37] "Taking to her bed," Lindberg writes, "was as easy as, or even easier than, breathing. Her un/conscious decision was one her spirit made. When it was time, and when the fury of her past began to race ahead of her future, she simply lay down."[38] The altered consciousness of the time spent in bed helps Bernice to process her trauma and to move forward with her life. In Shani Mootoo's *Cereus Blooms at Night*, Ambrose is so traumatized by the rape of his lover Mala that he sinks into endless slumber, waking only once a month to send packages of food to her. He spends many years this way, "cowering under a veil of sleep," until he finally awakes to an unrecognizable world.[39] In each of these novels, sleep, as a response to trauma, builds thematic weight as a profound symbolic figure of both suffering and endurance.

Nino Ricci's novel *Sleep* approaches the problem of excessive sleep differently – not as a response to trauma but as an intrinsic medical disorder. By focusing directly on disordered sleep (rather than using sleep as a figure for some other concern), the narrative finds a compelling way to establish the vital link between sleep and identity. If the conscious self depends on a regular pattern of restorative unconsciousness, the breakdown of predictable sleep brings about the destruction of the thoughts, feelings, and behaviours that constitute a persistent recognizable self. The protagonist of *Sleep*, historian David Pace, suffers from a disorder that causes him to fall asleep uncontrollably and unpredictably; in the opening scene, while David is driving on the highway with his young son Marcus in the back seat, sleep suddenly takes over his brain – "at once the urge is there, irresistible" – and he dozes off and nearly crashes at high speed.[40] David's disorder is never named, but it appears to be narcolepsy, with which Ricci himself has also been diagnosed.[41] As David loses the ability to stay awake, but refuses to reveal his condition to his family and colleagues out of a fear of vulnerability, he descends into anger, chaotic behaviour, and abuse of the various pharmaceuticals that he has been prescribed.

One of the cruelties of narcolepsy is that even though it brings about frequent sleeps, the sense of replenishment afforded by these sleeps tends to be limited or short-lived, and sufferers soon find themselves feeling sleepy all over again and at risk of dozing off in the middle of an activity.[42] In David's case, the disorder affects his notion of himself in two ways. First, the uncontrollable onset of multiple sleeps throughout the day means that he can no longer trust himself to live a fully independent life. Basic activities are suddenly hazardous, even when he is on his own, let alone when he is caring for Marcus. The nights are no safer, as David discovers that he has been carrying out unknown actions, even committing acts of violence, "in some middle state that is less sleep than waking dream."[43] In one heartbreaking scene, he fills his apartment with obstacles such as chairs, books, and masking tape when Marcus stays over, "in the hope of startling himself if he wanders."[44] David's inability to control his own behaviour and to live up to his responsibilities is a source of embarrassment and shame as well as danger. His sense that he has been condemned "to live in this place of constant incursion, where nothing was safe, nothing was certain,"[45] is thus a feeling that his own self has been taken away and twisted into something unrecognizable.

The inability to fulfill the expectations of adulthood thus brings about the second, closely related problem, as David finds that the lack of proper slumber short-circuits the ways that sleep is supposed to consolidate identity. He grimly claims that "the brain houses within its separate hemispheres actual warring consciousnesses ... [W]hat this means is that everyone carries within them a shadow self that dogs the dominant one like a stalker, always at odds, always seeking an outlet, awaiting its chance under cover of dark."[46] Sleep is a vital part of daily life, but it must be separated from wakefulness;

the dissolving of the boundary between the two throws the foundations of the mind into question.

Actual sleep scientists would likely see things a bit differently, although the implications of sleep for identity are indeed profound. Pioneering sleep researcher Rosalind D. Cartwright has observed that dreaming plays a key role in regulating emotions and in modifying the notion of the self; she asserts that "it is this 'self-system' which guides much of our waking behavior."[47] Sleep neurologist W. Chris Winter notes that disruptions to REM sleep can cause memory troubles as well as "attention problems, poor concentration, and potential mood disturbances."[48] Even if David's explanation of this process is not entirely scientific, he is acutely aware of how fragile his own identity has become. If one of the roles of sleep is to sort out which version of the self will rise to the surface of the waking mind, the impairment of this function means that David can no longer modulate his impulses or channel his thoughts into a state that aligns with coherent values. "Who knew," he wonders, "what mayhem threatened when the machinery faltered, at what point walking awake became as dangerous as asleep."[49] Without adequate sleep, the self becomes less recognizable, mutating into something more aggressive, violent, and unpredictable. Meanwhile, even though David's cocktail of medications may help with the more obvious symptoms, no drug can possibly reproduce the unfathomable function of sleep. The pills end up blurring the edges of the self even further, so that "who knew anymore what was him and what was the drugs taking him over."[50] As David spirals further into self-destructive behaviour, the failure of the synthetic regulation of consciousness through drugs only further emphasizes the irreplaceable position of sleep at the foundation of identity.

Sleep, unfortunately, is an unsatisfying novel, largely because David's chaotic behaviour ironically makes him too predictable. As literary scholar Kit Dobson puts it, "*Sleep* is deeply frustrating because David is so boneheaded."[51] The womanizing, gun-brandishing, pill-snorting history professor makes every possible worst decision, sabotaging the things that matter to him one by one: his marriage, his career, his relationship with his son, and in a cliffhanger ending, perhaps his own life. The novel never offers much sign of a compassionate or level-headed David, and we are left with the distinct impression that the narcolepsy can't take all the blame, that even a well-rested David would probably be just as self-destructive. (Bizarrely, many of the adult characters around him are also engaged in massively self-sabotaging behaviour despite their presumably unremarkable sleep.) Nevertheless, problems of character development aside, a key way that the novel develops a sense of interest is by investigating just how precariously the house of the waking mind rests on the shaky foundation of slumber. The idea that consciousness so crucially depends on sleep, that mysterious and fickle secret realm of the mind, can be deeply unsettling. Although *Sleep* does not explore its topic through any notable experimentation with literary form (in the manner of, say, *Wide Slumber for Lepidopterists*), it strikingly resists the all-too-common urge to see sleep merely as a trope, a figure, or even a form of healing from trauma. Sure, one could read sleep in Ricci's novel as a metaphor – as a comment on the flimsiness of self-regulation, for example, or on David's failure to remain alert to what is important in life – but a more memorable and harrowing reading comes about when we see David's sleep troubles as actual sleep troubles. Imperfect as it may be, *Sleep* seeks to directly confront the role of sleep in producing identity, leaving us to contemplate the stranger who might crawl out of bed in the morning if our sleep should go badly wrong.

Each work of fiction develops its own world of representation, and the above texts begin to hint at how novels can use the figures of deficient sleep, excessive sleep, unsettled sleep – and, every now and then, good restful sleep – to engage with many concerns, from the inequities of racism and sexism, to the burden of life choices, to the all-consuming nature of grief. Considering a variety of such works together as a cluster illuminates how visions of sleep can actively engage in the development of diverse forms of meaning, moving beyond the matter of "too much" sleep and "not enough." Sleep, these books reveal, cannot be limited to its function as a blank slate, an expression of passive innocence, or even a physical need. Rather, the place of sleep as a vital form of replenishment, as an unavoidable factor of human life, only amplifies its role as an active participant in the negotiation of meaning, identity, and power.

When it comes to fictions of sleep, the novel holds a special place in terms of sustained and thoughtful engagement, but other forms and genres also allow for fruitful investigation. Here, without attempting to undertake a comprehensive survey of all genres, I offer a look at one movie and one genre-defying book as examples of the possibilities that emerge from a wider variety of texts. *Awake* is an apocalyptic thriller that Canadian director Mark

Raso wrote with his brother Joseph Raso.[52] Produced by Netflix, the film portrays a mysterious global event that causes all electronic machinery to break down and deprives the entire human population of the ability to sleep. As their insomnia stretches on for days, the characters lose their grip on rational thought, eventually hallucinating, forming strange cults, and descending into violent paranoia. The protagonist, Jill Adams (Gina Rodriguez), comes to understand that everyone will die from sleep deprivation within a matter of days, and some of the movie's scenes are shot with a blurred focus as Jill loses her lucidity, her body slumping from exhaustion. In one scene, a scientist explains to Jill that a rogue solar flare is behind the sleep loss; the flare "changed our electromagnetic wiring. It affected our glymphatic system. Messed with our clocks." Jill's young daughter, Matilda (Ariana Greenblatt), who survives a near-drowning in the moments after the solar flare, miraculously still knows how to sleep, so the military captures her to try to extract a cure – a venture that ends when the soldiers at the medical hub lose their minds and all shoot one another. At the end of the movie, Matilda and her family discover that in order to relearn how to sleep, a person must die and be resuscitated through CPR, as this allows them to "start over."

Awake was lambasted by critics ("*Awake* will have audiences reaching for the snooze button," declared Rotten Tomatoes), but even if the film may not be a cinematic masterpiece, it reached number one in Netflix's global viewing rankings upon its release in June 2021.[53] For the millions of viewers who are already anxious about insomnia, a world without sleep makes for a terrifying and compelling premise. As cultural critic Simon Orpana says, "The apocalyptic fears of societal collapse that haunt and entice us by turns are symptoms of toxic realities, histories and relationships we are already immersed in."[54] Interestingly, a world without sleep also makes for a narrative that is nearly indistinguishable from a zombie flick: a mysterious infliction spreads throughout the population, turning normal people into mindless, violent automatons, while a few scruffy protagonists try to make their way to a safe location to find a cure that might not really exist. In both cases, the social cohesion that enables a sense of community belonging is destroyed, leaving behind only frightened individuals who must struggle for bare life without ever being allowed to rest.

Zombie movies are often seen as indictments of the mindless ravages of consumer capitalism. By replacing the narrative element of the zombie virus with that of insomnia, *Awake* hints at the idea that sleep loss, more than consumer culture, is at the heart of the neoliberal destruction of compassionate communities. Sleep loss *is* the disease that emerges from a culture that no longer knows how to function as a society, a disease that in turn further destroys any sense of social cohesion, creating a vicious cycle of exhaustion, isolation, and peril. The degree to which the movie achieves its own awareness of this interpretive possibility, however, is less clear. We might say that the solar flare is a narrative gimmick that offers a simplistic, external source for a complex problem – a source that ironically draws attention away from the cultural causes of widespread sleep loss by conjuring a phenomenon beyond human control and indeed beyond our planet. To adapt literary scholar Fredric Jameson's famous maxim that "it is easier to imagine the end of the world than the end of capitalism,"[55] *Awake* implies that it is easier to imagine a shockwave from outer space than it is to grapple with neoliberal capitalism, climate collapse, and the breakdown of social safety nets.

The "cure" that the characters discover, which requires stopping their own beating hearts, suggests that there is, in a sense, no way to redeem the sleepless society. The only way out is death, followed by the birth of something new. However, even this faint glimmer of rebirth at the end of the movie has already potentially been poisoned. Midway through the film, as the family makes their way in a repaired car down a hazardous, pitch-dark road through a forest, Jill has Matilda sit in the driver's seat, believing that Matilda will need to know how to drive when she is the family's only survivor. Dodge, an escaped convict riding in the back seat, says, "You know, my grandmama, you know what she used to tell me? That all the world's problems could all disappear in one generation if every kid grew up forgetting all the shit they were taught, the shit that doesn't make sense, but you're taught it enough times, you believe it. Then we can actually live in a world where no one is starving and everyone's equal." Matilda, her tiny hands gripping the steering wheel, turns all the way around to look at Dodge, and asks, "Really?" – causing the car to swerve and nearly veer off the road until Jill frantically reaches for the wheel and corrects the course. This little vignette ambivalently suggests that even if a new world is possible, the young generation who can bring it forth does not know how to steer. Whatever new world emerges from the ashes of this one will also face the risk of running off the road and tumbling down the embankment of sleep loss.

With all electronics rendered useless by the solar flare, it is the loss of automobiles that resonates most deeply throughout the film. That the disaster causes the breakdown of both sleep and cars (a seemingly strange pair) hints at the vital position of cars, and thus fossil fuels, in the psyche of modern culture, as though the safety and replenishment afforded by sleep can't survive if the characters can't fire up the engine and go for a drive. Jill's theft of a rare functioning vehicle – a 1972 Dodge Polara, old enough to be relatively free of modern electronics – is a major victory for her family in their search for the ability to sleep. The crucial role of cars in the movie lends a special significance to the scene where Dodge, who shares his name with the car, sits in the back seat dreaming about a utopian future, only to have Matilda nearly crash the vehicle. Dodge's vision of a world where everyone is equal emerges while he slouches in the moving car, as though the vehicle powers his memory of his grandmother and his ability to imagine a brighter future. As his name suggests, there is a sense in which he *is* the car, in that his subjectivity is tied to its reassuring forward motion. The Polara carries its passengers toward the medical hub, where they hope to regain their sleep, and it also fuels their hopeful vision of a new world. The vehicle and its repaired combustion engine seductively seem to enable the peace of mind and fertility of imagination necessary for good sleep and hope, yet the car, as a symbol of consumer capitalism, fossil fuels, and ecological collapse, is a dangerous machine that threatens to crash and kill them all. If the characters are unable to envision a reborn world that doesn't reproduce the mentality of consumption and extraction tied to automobile culture, what hope do they have of freeing themselves of the cultural forces behind systemic sleep loss? Jill and her family may restore their ability to sleep at the end of the story, but the movie hints that the characters might use the power of sleep only to recreate the insomniac world their imaginations cannot escape.

Another way of looking at how *Awake* juxtaposes the breakdown of cars with the breakdown of sleep is to say that by forcing the characters to quit the habit of fossil fuels, the solar flare (a burst of renewable solar energy) causes them to "wake up" from what Orpana would call the acquiescent slumber of petroculture. However, this awakening is a cruel one, as the world to which the characters must bear witness in their exhaustion is a violent, paranoid place. Orpana's thesis in his book *Gasoline Dreams: Waking Up from Petroculture*, that moving beyond fossil fuels requires an immensely difficult cultural shift of collective imagination, usefully illuminates why the characters in *Awake* cling so desperately to the last fragments of the petroleum-powered world. As Orpana says about the postapocalyptic thriller *A Quiet Place* (another movie where a disastrous event stops the characters from using fossil fuels),[56] "such fantasies engage our desires for change while negotiating with our fears of the unknown, thus retrenching the same old paradigms."[57] We might also turn to the work of political scientist Cara New Daggett in her book *The Birth of Energy*, where she argues that switching from fossil energy to clean energy is not enough to save us, that "we need new energy figures and metaphors, and new ways of valuing energetic activity."[58] *Awake* shows us a world where the loss of one "energy figure" – combustion cars – coincides with the loss of vibrant human life as exhaustion overtakes the sleepless protagonists. However, no *new* energy figure is proposed, and the characters scramble desperately to restore the old ones. The challenge posed by this narrative, then, is the matter of how we might decouple two key energy figures; how can we sleep well and replenish our bodies without holding on to the capitalist vision of extractive productivity?

Whether the "intention" of *Awake* is to critique petroculture, or whether the movie, like its characters, is too entangled in petroculture to see very far beyond it, is perhaps not the most interesting question. Rather, by linking the breakdown of sleep with the breakdown of cars and other technologies, the movie inspires us to ask ourselves how we relate to the insomniac world of modern culture and whether the path toward good sleep involves keeping the Dodge running at all costs or imagining radically changed forms of energy and social relations. *Awake*, then, is a story about whether it is possible to enjoy good sleep in the Anthropocene, a problem to which I return in chapter 5.

Suzanne Buffam's *A Pillow Book* is a strange little volume that refuses to be categorized as memoir, fiction, or essay. The original *Pillow Book* was a collection of observations and private musings, a sort of rambling diary, written by Sei Shōnagon in the court of Empress Teishi in Japan around the year 1000.[59] Whereas the original volume, which Buffam describes as "an exhaustive catalogue of petty grievances,"[60] did not actually take pillows as its subject, Buffam's book develops a sustained and playful interest in this most intimate sleep accessory, serving as an informal cultural inquiry into the often overlooked role that pillows play within our lives. Her book is a kind of love letter to the pillow, and, much like a poem, it asks us to see a familiar object in surprising new terms.

A pillow can easily be said to symbolize sleep (often doing so in sleep product ads), and Buffam notes that "by the time we die, most of us will have spent a quarter of a century adrift on our pillows."[61] Yet this long-term relationship with the pillow happens largely out of sight even for the participant, as the dissolution of consciousness during sleep means that, for the most part, a person's lengthy and intimate partnership with their pillow cannot be experienced directly. "We know less about what happens on our pillows at night," Buffam writes, "than we know about the dark side of the moon."[62] She is referring to the limitations of scientific knowledge about the role of sleep in human health, although the comment could just as easily hint at the slipperiness of direct experience of sleep. Our profound relationship with pillows, then, tends to be vastly underacknowledged, as is confirmed by the fact that a book about a person's relationship with her pillow likely seems frivolous at first glance (literary scholars have had no apparent interest in *A Pillow Book*). The last line of the book – "If you want to go to sleep, kiss your pillow goodnight"[63] – presents the pillow as a sleep partner or a lover, a figure of companionship with an agency of its own. This comment is perhaps reminiscent of Marie Kondo's advice in her extraordinarily popular book *The Life-Changing Magic of Tidying Up*, where she instructs her readers to thank each item of clothing and each household possession for its service to their life and to "greet your house every time you come home."[64] For readers who would normally feel no sense of allegiance to the animistic notion of entering into relationship with the energies or intentions of everyday objects, these acts are startling defamiliarizations, yet the perspective afforded by greeting your house or kissing your pillow is in some way self-evident in its recognition that objects are significant for how they shape the character of lived experience.

Unlike Kondo's book, however, *A Pillow Book* is full of irony, self-doubt, and exasperation. Much of Buffam's interest in pillows emerges from her own painful insomnia. (Should we say "the speaker," rather than Buffam? The nature of the narrative persona is unclear.) "I have the sleep hygiene of a narcoleptic truck-driver on crank, I learn on my pillow by my phone's blue glow," she writes. "My failure is moral, as much as it is physiological."[65] Her sleeplessness means that she spends a great deal of conscious time resting on her pillow, with the result that her relationship with her pillow becomes, in a sense, more obvious and noteworthy than that of a good sleeper. Many of the snippets of narrative in the book recall waking moments that have happened in the company of her pillow, such as watching her husband's sleeping form, listening to her young daughter explain why she needs to get out of bed, or lying awake during her own childhood with a flashlight and a box of Trivial Pursuit cards.[66] The pillow thus becomes the companion or accessory of insomnia even more than it is an accessory of sleep. The final line of the book, "If you want to go to sleep, kiss your pillow goodnight," is thus the dubious advice of a failed practitioner.

Although many of Buffam's observations might ring philosophical or indeed strike one as a catalogue of petty grievances, *A Pillow Book* soon reveals that talking about pillows also means talking about cultural politics. The tentacles of consumer culture reach deeply into Buffam's bedroom. There, she wakes at 3:00 a.m. and then fails to sleep for the rest of the night while watching "the one hundred and one worst red carpet disasters of all time." Or she tries out insomnia remedies one after another, none of which work, from melatonin and Lunesta to a comical variety of luxury pillows, including (among many others) "the Brookstone Biosense Memory Foam Shoulder Pillow," "the Viscofresh Advanced Contour Memory Foam Classic Pillow," and "the Sobakawa Cloud, as seen on TV, with over thirty million cooling micro-air beads to conform to my shoulders and neck, while cradling my head in a fluffy cloud of nanotechnology."[67] Each specialty pillow is made ironic by its own self-important name and by its inclusion in the absurdly lengthy list of nearly identical products. Nevertheless, Buffam obsesses over these consumer sleep aids, and understandably so; these pillows turn sleep from an untroubled bodily act into a high-tech endeavour requiring expertise, status, and the discerning eye of a skilled shopper. When Buffam chastises herself for her "moral" failure after her smartphone tells her that she has poor sleep hygiene, we see how her own relationship with sleep has become deeply intertwined with the ideologies of neoliberal self-sufficiency and mass consumption. A pillow is not just a pillow; it is an emblem that testifies to a person's virtue, intelligence, and economic and social positions.

Like other discourses on sleep and its accoutrements, then, *A Pillow Book* is not just about pillows, beds, or the sleeping that takes place on them. Investigating the material objects tied to sleep also involves thinking about the cultural values attached to these objects and about the visions of hope, inadequacy, and meaning that they conjure, whether consciously or not. "In all the innumerable galleries throughout the art museums of the world," Buffam writes, "it is hard to find one featuring a pillow that does not also squeeze in a young woman's breast."[68] The pillow has always been co-opted through association with other desires and forms of power, all too often tied to the matter of whose voices are heard and whose are silenced – whose works of art, whose works of writing, whose product ads and smartphone apps are granted the brightest spotlight on the cultural stage. Working to understand the role of the pillow in our lives may involve kissing our pillow goodnight, but it also requires building a critical literacy of cultural visions of sleep.

We could examine any number of additional texts for insights into the representation of sleep in narrative fiction and other forms. A person could develop a detailed study of the significance of sleep in, for instance, Dionne Brand's novel *In Another Place, Not Here,* which traces the often sleepless lives of two women in the African Caribbean diaspora. Sleep can serve as a figure of indoctrination into the responsibilities of adulthood, as when Marilla, the adoptive mother in Lucy Maud Montgomery's novel *Anne of Green Gables,* admonishes Anne for the frivolity of wanting to decorate her bedroom with maple branches, telling her, "Bedrooms were made to sleep in."[69] And sleep can take material form through memorable images beyond pillows, such as the image of Jared's sleeping bag in Eden Robinson's novel *Son of a Trickster.* As Jared tries to complete high school while enduring family violence, drug addictions, and other repercussions of colonization, he retreats repeatedly to the sleeping bag in his basement bedroom, only to find that even this symbol of refuge is powerless to protect him from the troubles that saturate his world. In Canada and elsewhere, fictions of sleep open into a rich world of aesthetic astonishment and political acumen, allowing us to build a more informed and subtle imaginative vision of those all-too-often invisible hours of the night when awareness ostensibly melts away.

THE THEFT OF DREAMS IN *THE MARROW THIEVES*

The matter of dreams has not been my central concern in this book because I am primarily interested in uncovering the functions of sleep that tend to be less recognized or visible, but I close this chapter with a consideration of the work that dreams can do within literary fiction. The close relationship between sleep and dreams allows for rich possibilities in terms of imaginative representation. On a figurative level, the notion of the dream is the ultimate cliché for a hopeful vision of the future and for the aspiration to bring about positive change. Literature – which might be called a series of daydreams in published form or, more ambitiously, the embodiment of the grand dreams of a society – has a more obvious historical and conceptual relationship with dreams than it necessarily does with sleep. Drawing on comments from Argentine writer Jorge Luis Borges, literary scholar Peter Schwenger has elaborated at length on the notion that "literature is nothing more than a guided dream."[70] Every book – resting, as it were, under its covers – carries out a silent dream life. Much of the discussion about literature and dreams can paradoxically move rather far away from my concern with sleep, so rather than diving into the deep and murky waters of literature as it relates to dreams in general, I look more specifically at an example of a close literary link between dreams and sleep – in this case, one that operates in terms of cultural politics and Indigenous representation.

Cherie Dimaline's novel *The Marrow Thieves*, which won the Governor General's Award for children's literature in 2017 and was a Canada Reads contender in 2018, is a dystopian story that takes place in the second half of the twenty-first century. Dimaline, a Métis writer, develops an imaginative future that reflects ecological destruction as well as the concerns of violent colonization in Canada; the story builds a link between the history of the residential schools and the possibility of future colonial violence that may yet unfold as the settler society crumbles in the face of climate collapse. That the book can be said to straddle the boundary between young adult fiction and adult fiction has allowed it to reach a wide audience, and the book has become a particularly notable work of recent Indigenous literature, selling over 100,000 copies in Canada, with a sequel published in 2021 and a television series in the works.[71] The notion of dreams figures prominently in the novel and becomes intertwined with the necessary and problematic act of sleeping, such that sleep and dreams are key elements in the representation of colonization and its associated harms.

The narrator of *The Marrow Thieves* is Frenchie, a Métis youth on the run from the villainous Recruiters, who kidnap Indigenous people and take them to government-run facilities where scientists harvest their bone marrow, the part of the body that is said to allow for the ability to dream. Frenchie joins a small group of Cree, Métis, and Anishinaabe survivors who are living together in a forest north of what used to be Toronto, and the bulk of the story involves their efforts to move from camp to camp in order to avoid capture as they make their way farther north.

Because the narrative is focused on the Indigenous characters, the state of the settler society is mostly revealed indirectly through exposition, yet the settlers' motivation is key to the unfolding events. The settler society has collapsed as a result of the climate crisis. Coastlines are unrecognizable, the Arctic has undergone extensive melting, California has been submerged, wars have been fought over fresh water supplies, and half the population has died from disaster and disease. Torrential rains flood the land, pollinating insects and most wildlife have vanished, and crumbling cities have been abandoned. Faced with a profound sense of guilt, the survivors have lost the ability to dream and to sleep well.

Dreams operate here in a relatively literal sense as well as in a more figurative sense. When the settlers lose the literal ability to dream, they enter "a plague of madness," an "insanity that crept like bedbugs through families while they slept."[72] Miig, the leader of Frenchie's group, explains that "people lost their minds, killing themselves and others."[73] Frenchie pictures the dying settlers "just shutting off like factory machines at the end of a shift."[74] Even if the loss of sleep and dreams operates as a conceit of the dystopian fiction, the resulting madness involves a certain degree of logic; as I mentioned in my discussion of Nino Ricci's *Sleep*, REM sleep and dreams are vital for sustaining emotional and mental health and ultimately for producing and modifying one's sense of self.

Of course, the functioning of sleep and dreams on a "literal" level (always a risky word) leads immediately into more figurative and even allegorical realms. The settlers' insomnia and the destruction of their ability to "dream" – that is, their capacity to foster hope, meaning, purpose, and vision for the future – emphasize the torture that they must endure and also reflect their profound guilt, as they must live with their legacy of ecosystem collapse, disease, and the destruction of their society. As Frenchie explains to young RiRi, "with all this sickness and movement and death, people got sad. One of the ways the sadness came out was when they slept. They stopped being able to dream ... They visited their head doctors – psychiatrists – and they took pills to help them sleep when they stopped having the will to lie down at night. Soon they turned on each other, and the world changed again."[75] The settlers' response to insomnia involves searching for solutions in the consumer pharmaceutical industry and Western medicine, individualistic approaches that avoid facing up to systemic acts of destruction and the resulting guilt. This sense of trust in science and technology to solve what is really an ethical or spiritual problem – a notion that reflects the sociological link between the medicalization of sleep and its commodification – foreshadows the monstrous technology that will be used to steal Indigenous dreams.[76]

Rather than trying to atone in some way for what they have done, the settlers double down on the infliction of violence, creating a new version of the residential school system in the form of facilities where Indigenous people are killed to create a dream elixir for the settler population (although the story is never clear about whether this remedy actually works). The theft of dreams is thus the re-enactment, or rather the continuation, of the worst atrocities of colonization. The Recruiters who hunt the Indigenous survivors are in fact "school truancy officers" working for the Government of Canada in the "Department of Oneirology."[77] Oneirology is the scientific study of dreams, and the name of the department is Orwellian in the sense that its true function is to steal and thus destroy dreams. Sound sleep becomes a grotesque form of currency, and the implication of the settlers' plight is that the more dreams they try to steal, the more dreams they will lose.[78]

Although the novel critiques the settlers' violent commodification of sleep, it also invites readings informed by Indigenous understandings of the significance of dreams. Such accounts are diverse, but Indigenous writers have often identified important connections between dreaming and the cultural structures of identity, knowledge, and spirit. In her study of Anishinaabe ways of learning, Leanne Betasamosake Simpson writes, "Knowledge is often transmitted from the spiritual world to humans through dreaming and visioning."[79] She observes that problems can be solved and choices clarified during sleep. In his essay "On Native Mythology," Cree author Tomson Highway writes, "The mythology of a people is the articulation of the dreamworld of that people; without that dreamlife being active in all its forms – from the most extreme beauty to the most horrific and back – the culture of that people is dead. It is a dead culture and it is, in effect, a dead people we speak of."[80] Willie Ermine, a scholar from the Sturgeon Lake First Nation in Saskatchewan who is known in particular for his development of the notion of the "ethical space," sees dreams as a central element of Indigenous epistemology.

He notes that the spirit, which is a key point of access for knowledge, "is the haven of dreams, those peculiar images that flash symbolic messages to the knower. Dreams are the link to the spiritual world from whence our spirit comes ... Our progenitors knew and believed in the power of dreams; it is only through dreams that sacred undertakings are attempted. Blessings and other assorted gifts that permeate Aboriginal thought all stem from dreams."[81]

Indigenous literature in Canada has sometimes echoed these thoughts, the best-known example probably being the starting point for mischievous creation on the first page of Thomas King's *Green Grass, Running Water*, where the storyteller says, "Coyote was there, but Coyote was asleep. That Coyote was asleep and that Coyote was dreaming. When that Coyote dreams, anything can happen."[82] Within the larger context from which such representations draw – where dreams serve as a foundation for culture, stories, and knowledge – the ability of the Indigenous characters in *The Marrow Thieves* to dream implies a continuation of Indigenous ways of life, in contrast to the settler society's collapse into a dead culture. In a sense, the novel poses a conflict between two cultural models of sleep and dreams. The survival of Indigenous sleep signifies the survival of the Indigenous worldviews, and the disappearance of settler sleep represents the near extinction of the medical-technological and Christian worldviews, the latter being kept on life support by the scientists and church officials in the residential schools.

In Dimaline's novel, a striking feature of the collapse of the settler society amidst violence and disease is the way that it echoes the earlier near collapse of Indigenous societies amidst colonization. Several scholars have shown that for Indigenous communities living within a history of colonization, the apocalypse, in a very real sense, has already happened. Philosopher and environmental justice scholar Kyle Powys Whyte notes that due to the colonial attacks on ecosystems and ways of life, "Anishinaabek already inhabit what our ancestors would have understood as a dystopian future."[83] The project of colonization has attempted to sweep Indigenous societies away, leaving behind dead cultures, and in this sense the residential school system was always in the business of stealing dreams. In Dimaline's imagined future, the settlers now experience their own apocalypse and the loss of their individual and collective dreams.[84]

The Marrow Thieves contains a few scenes where the Indigenous characters encounter their own troubles with sleep, and these temporary breakages tend to highlight the conditions of community and good faith that are necessary for peaceful sleep and dreams. In one key scene, Frenchie's group comes across an abandoned tourist hotel called the Four Winds Resort. Here, rather than sleeping as usual in a group camp, each character takes a separate room. "It was strange," Frenchie observes, "all of us separated by walls."[85] Soon, Frenchie's love interest, Rose, comes to join him in his bed, but they are interrupted when young RiRi also comes into the room, asking to sleep with them. Then their friend Slopper appears, saying, "Move over, French. I can't sleep."[86] When Frenchie wakes up the next morning, Minerva, the Elder, is sitting in a chair in the room, Chi-Boy and Wab are sleeping on the floor, Miig is leaning against the wall, and Frenchie's feet are "trapped under a weight on top of the blankets that turned out to be Tree and Zheegwon lying perpendicular on top of the comforter."[87] The comical scene indicates that good sleep for these characters is communal, and that the settler emphasis on individuality signified by the solitary rooms of the tourist resort is hostile to the conditions of group togetherness that enable successful slumber. The most mundane elements of the settler world – rooms with walls and doors and separate beds – are designed in a way that makes sleep difficult for the Indigenous characters; the scene ironizes the settler approach to sleep simply through an encounter with architecture. This assessment is not meant to imply that communal sleep is "better" than sleeping in separate rooms but that the Indigenous characters must rework the settler infrastructure to find the sleep practice that works for them.[88]

More ominously, both Frenchie and Miig commit acts of violence in the novel, and as a result, both temporarily lose the ability to sleep or dream. After killing a man whose betrayal has resulted in the death of RiRi, Frenchie is overcome with guilt: "I fell into dreamless sleep with a throb and a pull in my body."[89] Miig, meanwhile, relates a story about his encounter with an employee of the residential schools. Even though the man is "just a cog in the system," Miig shoots him and leaves him for dead on a remote road.[90] "He pleaded with me to take him," Miig says, "but I was deaf to him then. Not that I wouldn't hear him clearly later when I tried to sleep."[91] Frenchie and Miig thus come dangerously close to the settler experience that is so monstrous in the novel, emphasizing the risk of succumbing to violence and the need to maintain good spiritual standing.

Ultimately, the ability of the Indigenous protagonists to continue to dream is tied to the recovery and renewal of cultural knowledge. The extraction technology in one of the residential schools breaks down when Minerva, who is hooked up to the machines, sings traditional songs in the Anishinaabemowin language. "As it turns out," Frenchie says, "every dream Minerva had ever dreamed was in the language. It was her gift, her secret, her plan."[92] The language contains the dreams, and as Frenchie learns, the dreams contain the language; the Cree characters dream in their language, Nehiyawok.[93] A story that seems to be about the settlers' theft of dreams turns out largely to be about the positive work of strengthening the languages and traditional forms of knowledge that are tied to the ability to dream.

Benjamin Reiss argues that the crisis of sleep in modern society is in fact two crises: "a psychological struggle, in which those who live in relative states of comfort try to wrestle their sleep into submission, and a more existential struggle experienced by those who are expected to sleep by the rules of others yet are denied the time, space, and security to do so. What links these two sets of struggles is the growing economization of sleep."[94] Dimaline's dystopia takes the economization of sleep to an extreme, where sleep becomes a commodity that is extracted without permission, creating an existential struggle for Indigenous dreams, life, and culture. However, by imagining this problem as a conflict between two cultural models of sleep, the novel emphasizes how one response to the crisis that arises when sleep comes under assault can hinge not on trying to gain the security to sleep "by the rules of others" but on reclaiming an independent model of sleep that exists outside of the culturally dominant one.

INTERLUDE

Sleeping through Covid-19

THE COVID-19 PANDEMIC, especially the sudden lockdowns throughout most of the world in early 2020, can illuminate some of the key issues at stake in how sleep operates as both practice and representation – as both a bodily need tied to social concerns and a form of manipulation and power. In the most literal terms, the pandemic created widespread problems with sleep loss, emphasizing how sleep can be a key measure of inequity and public health. In more conceptual terms, the pandemic became an unexpected battlefield for conflicting visions of sleep as a figure of differing values in a time when some of the most basic foundations of social structures were destabilized. The pandemic gives us a lesson in how the ability to read sleep critically is a vital skill for sorting through contested visions of the social sphere.

As the SARS-COV-2 virus that causes Covid-19, and the restrictive social measures meant to counter its transmission, spread across the globe during the first few months of 2020, sleep was profoundly disrupted for vast numbers of people. In part, the experience of sleep became tied up with the larger disruptions to the usual structuring of time. The routine of daily schedules fell apart as people had to stay home from their jobs, their classrooms, their parties, restaurants, and even walks in the park. The hours of the clock lost some of their meaning, and sleep was one of many daily events whose character was profoundly altered.

However, these effects rippled through society in very unequal ways. People working from home may have had to attend video calls from their bedrooms, suddenly broadcasting a public view of their intimate sleeping quarters.[1] For parents of young children, the internal family structure of sleep may have formed new rhythms, cut loose from the demands of work schedules and classrooms. Many parents, mostly women, had to spend their daytime hours supervising home schooling, leaving them to catch up on their "day" jobs at night, sacrificing sleep along the way. A study in 2020 found "levels of sleep deprivation in moms that were twice as high as those seen before the pandemic" – a situation that in some cases persisted for years.[2] Racial disparities, which had already been implicated in sleep loss, were also exacerbated by the pandemic.[3] For people who were suddenly unemployed, the alarm clock may no longer have structured sleep in predictable ways, and for those whose jobs were deemed essential – disproportionately women and people of colour – daily routines may have remained intact but were carried out under the shadow of constant physical danger and anxious nights.[4]

As the stress and isolation dragged on, pandemic-related nightmares drew widespread attention through the social media hashtags #pandemicdreams and #covidnightmares, with sleepers recounting dreams about "getting lost in a crowd of people who constantly bump into you and spread their germs," "being attacked while trying to buy sanitizer," or "arriving late for an important Zoom video chat meeting."[5] One study found that the nightmares and other sleep disruptions among people in Italy were consistent with those of post-traumatic stress disorder.[6] Just like earthquake survivors, who tend to have more severe nightmares the closer they were to the epicentre, the people at the front lines of the pandemic reported the closest encounters with the terrors of the night.[7] Atul Khullar, an Edmonton sleep clinic consultant, commented that the stress of the pandemic – caused by fear of the virus itself as well as the sudden loss of daily structure – was exacerbating the problem of insomnia in those who already suffered from it and was creating new bouts of sleeplessness in others.[8] Remaining vigilant at night is an evolutionary survival technique triggered by fear, but as the pandemic stretched from days to weeks to years, the continuous anxiety took a severe toll on the population.[9] Neurologists started to speak of "COVID-somnia."[10] The use of sleeping pills soared worldwide.[11] Social divisiveness around public health restrictions also caused sleep loss, as when insurgents in the so-called Freedom Convoy in Ottawa in 2022 blared air horns capable of causing permanent hearing damage for eleven straight nights until a judge granted an injunction.[12]

In contrast, some people found that their sleep habits improved or that they usefully adapted them during the lockdowns. With the sudden transition to working from home, many employees found that the hours that otherwise would have been spent commuting were now freed up for other activities, including getting more sleep.[13] Teenagers had the chance to develop a new relationship with sleep when school closures moved their studies online. With some schools abandoning daytime class schedules, studying became asynchronous, meaning that students could log in and complete their work at whatever time of day was most convenient. As a result, some teenagers switched to nocturnal patterns, sleeping during the day and carrying out their studies and socializing online at night.[14] This desynchronization of sleep, during which different family members in the same household would meet one another occasionally on the way to and from their beds, allowed young people, whose social and biological needs may differ from those of their parents, to reimagine daily time in a way that was previously impossible.

Among people who caught Covid, sleep loss became an unexpected problem in another way, as insomnia turned out to be one of the most common long-haul symptoms of the disease.[15] Rachel Salas, a neurologist at Johns Hopkins University, commented that the sleep disturbances seen during the first waves of the pandemic were likely "just the beginning of long-term effects we're going to see for years to come."[16] Other Covid sufferers, meanwhile, found themselves afflicted with overwhelming exhaustion and perpetual sleepiness, with no amount of slumber able to reduce the endless fatigue.[17] This certainly characterized my own experience with Covid during the Omicron wave of 2022. Prior to Covid, I had never been able to understand how some people are able to lie down and travel to dreamland in a few minutes. Falling asleep in anything less than half an hour was a concept foreign to me. After I caught Covid for the first time, that all changed. Everyday tasks such as making breakfast or reading a document would fill me with an overpowering sense of not only tiredness but also actual sleepiness. I found that I could stagger into the bedroom in the middle of the day and fall immediately asleep. I had finally learned how to nap, only to discover that I was better off without this particular skill. Luckily, my sleepiness faded away within a few weeks rather than turning into a case of long Covid.

All of these scenarios show how disruptions to sleep both reflect and contribute to changes in larger patterns of time use, work, public health, and daily life. That the changes to sleep patterns during the pandemic were not just sudden and drastic but also diverse and uneven emphasizes how sleep is contingent on social and health conditions that are always unequally felt. Many people have observed that the pandemic, although global in scale, impacted people inequitably, and experiences with sleep are a key way that these differences can be understood. Moreover, diverse encounters with sleep can reflect changing conditions over time; the people who enjoyed more sleep during the lockdowns and those who suffered alarming disruptions to their sleep may sometimes have been the same people, just at different stages of the arduous ebbs and flows of life in a radically changed world.

The significance of sleep always expands beyond the realm of literal slumber, and sure enough, figurative representations of sleep during the Covid lockdowns reflected and shaped vital forms of influence and value. In response to the widespread sleeplessness during the pandemic, BBC Radio broadcast a performance of "Sleep," a unique piece of classical music by British composer Max Richter. Described as an "eight-hour lullaby" originally performed over the course of a night in September 2015 for a live audience of sleeping listeners, "Sleep" holds the record for "the longest single continuous music broadcast the BBC has ever made."[18] Pointing to the apparently universal concept of the lullaby, Richter observes that sleep and music "seem to be related altered states."[19] His composition is meant to encourage slow reflection and to prompt subconscious engagement with music during the act of sleeping. In rebroadcasting this "lullaby for a frenetic world" during the initial Covid lockdown, the BBC noted that the music "offers a mindful way to forget everything going on around us and to enter another world."[20] This broadcast, which aired simultaneously across Europe through the European Broadcasting Union, represents the act of sleeping as both a threatened practice and an act of resistance and escape. Whereas the pandemic led to a widespread assault on the practice of sleeping, Richter's composition grants sleep a form of agency, or at least a tangible expression through art, that allows it to push back against the anxieties that keep people awake. By transforming the literal act of sleeping into representation through music, the composition hopes to provide its listeners with a talisman of mindfulness that they can take back with them into a restful night. Ironically, it is by taking sleep from practice to representation that the music intends to alter the actual experience of sleep.

Whereas Richter's "Sleep" engages directly with the practice of sleeping, other representations of sleep during the lockdowns relied on entirely figurative visions of sleep. The sense that the social world was slowing down, or even grinding to a halt, invited metaphors about the world entering a period of sleep, in the sense of inactivity, waiting, and the anticipation of new opportunities. Importantly, these envisioned future opportunities were not universal or neutral but reflected competing forms of value. Writing about the need for society to embrace the lessons of the pandemic, public policy economist Dennis Snower commented that "once the crisis is over, we will hopefully awaken into a new world."[21] This metaphor of awakening frames the present as a time of dormancy, of unawareness, that can be regarded with irony even while still underway. We are asked to see ourselves as enduring a period of sleep from which we must work hard to emerge so that society can become active and intelligent "once we have awoken to the new economic realities."[22] What the nature of these new realities might be and whether they should really be approached primarily through the lens of economics remain open questions, but whatever the specific priorities, this vision of sleep seeks to prepare us for transformation, for a new form of consciousness adapted to a changed world.

Closely linked to metaphors of sleep, the image of society undergoing a period of dormancy (from the Latin *dormire*, meaning "to sleep") appeared in various forms, and these images, too, reflected specific sets of values. A news report in the *Daily Mail* in the United Kingdom referred the viewer to a video showing "dozens of planes sitting dormant on a runway as airlines struggle to fill seats amid the coronavirus pandemic."[23] The phrasing is an uncanny echo of Emily St John Mandel's postapocalyptic pandemic-virus novel *Station Eleven*, in which abandoned jetliners "stood dormant on runways and in hangars. They collected snow on their wings."[24] However, whereas Snower's notion of awakening into a new world uses the image of sleep as a figure of hopeful transformation, the report about the airplanes portrays the dormancy of the transportation infrastructure as a form of brokenness, a state of damage from which the industry must try to recover. Caught up in these diverging figures of sleep is the tension between the desire to "return" to pre-pandemic life and the desire to embrace inevitable change.

Indeed, the matter of getting "back to normal" became a flashpoint of debate during the pandemic. Many people understandably craved a return to a familiar world without lockdowns, masks, and daily fears about a new virus, whereas others pointed to the terrors that had already pervaded that familiar world, from systemic poverty to rampant carbon emissions, and saw in the pandemic a chance to transform society. Dionne Brand, former poet laureate of Toronto, argued in the *Toronto Star* that returning to normal should not be the goal:

> Was the violence against women normal? Was the anti-Black and anti-Indigenous racism normal? Was white supremacy normal? Was the homelessness growing on the streets normal? Were homophobia and transphobia normal? Were pervasive surveillance and policing of Black and Indigenous and people of colour normal? Yes, I suppose all of that was normal. But, I and many other people hate that normal. Who would one have to be to sit in that normal restfully, to mourn it, or to desire its continuance?[25]

A similar frustration was visible in Toronto in 2021 when youth climate activists, calling for stronger action against greenhouse gas emissions, held up a banner that read, "We're not going back to normal."[26] The wish to return to normal, so frequently expressed, was not a neutral aspiration but one that reflected an investment in particular configurations of power. Jason Farman, a media scholar who studies the politics of waiting, also noted that the common narrative about "waking up" and getting back to normal was a "damaging way of thinking about 2020, because it erases it, rather than saying that this has been a year of tremendous learning and transition."[27] The experience of waiting, Farman argues, creates the opportunity to question our values and hopes.

A series of advertisements from Mazda Canada, which aired on television and online during the lockdown of spring 2020, shows how the figure of sleep can play a key role in this kind of cultural debate. The ads promote the seductive power of the desire to return to what is familiar, an impulse that is expressed through an image of sleep that frames the lockdown as a pause from normal daily life. Reading sleep carefully in these ads can foster the critical skills necessary for responding to the ideological visions embedded within images of slumber across texts and media of all kinds.

An ad titled "Sleeping Roads," which formed the centrepiece of the Mazda campaign, consists of a series of slowly panning shots of empty, silent roads

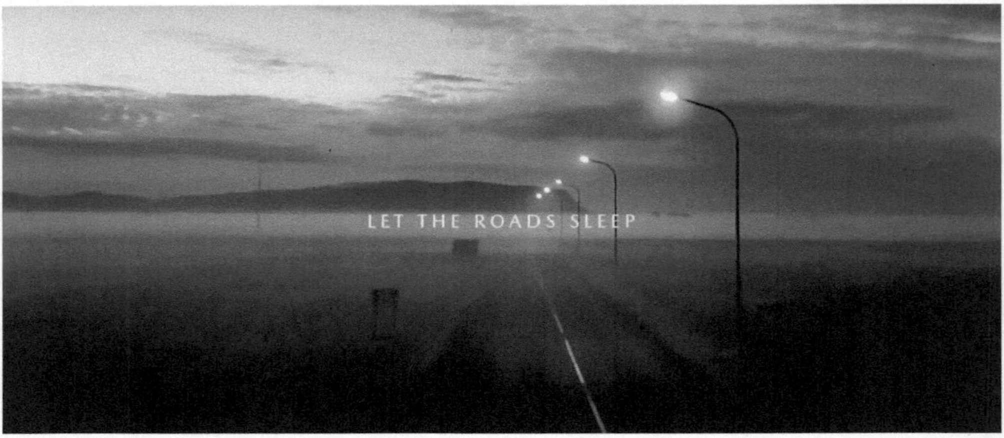

I.1 Mazda Canada, "Sleeping Roads," 2020.

at night.[28] Shot from an elevated height, the scenes develop a dreamy, nostalgic perspective as the viewer glides slowly forward along abandoned roads, passing a strip of restaurants, a suburban row of houses, and a vast plain with mountains in the distance. Each of these scenes is presented in near darkness, with ghostly streetlights faintly illuminating the empty roads. Although it does not mention Covid outright, the ad is clearly about the pandemic lockdown. A hint of twilight in the otherwise darkened skies sets the scenes ambiguously either at dusk or just before dawn, simultaneously representing the ending of one day and the beginning of a new one. Near the end of these scenes of darkness, a white tagline appears in the centre of the screen: "Let the roads sleep." In the final landscape to appear, a curved highway snakes through a low mountain pass alongside a lush forested coastline as waves lap at the distant shore. In this scene, the sun has now risen above the horizon, and a new dawn illuminates the road and the landscape. The overlaid message now concludes, "Because when they wake, we'll have a lot of catching up to do."

Whereas various cultural commentators during the lockdown asserted that life would never exactly return to the way it used to be prior to Covid-19, the Mazda ad deploys the sleep metaphor to portray the pandemic as merely a temporary interruption to the normal, seemingly timeless state of automobile culture. By resisting the notion that the world is undergoing a transformation, the ad primes its audience to anticipate the moment when the comforts of consumer culture will simply pick up where they left off. The notion that "we'll have a lot of catching up to do" implies that viewers are building up a deficit of driving, a debt that will need to be repaid by spending more time on the roads once they wake up.[29] By portraying the road as an old friend, as someone we will need to catch up with once the lockdown has ended, the ad also plays to the sense of isolation that many people had to endure during the strictest phases of social distancing. When the lockdown is over, this ad assures us, old friendships will emerge from their slumber, not least of which is your friendship with your Mazda.

The ad's soundtrack is a slow, mournful acoustic cover of the 1961 Ben E. King classic "Stand by Me," performed by American singer Skylar Grey. "When the night has come," she sings, "and the land is dark, and the moon is the only light we'll see ..." That is as far as she gets before the ad reaches the end of its fifteen-second runtime. Like the notion of sleep as a temporary state of waiting in anticipation of a new dawn, the incomplete lyric about the night and the moon places us within darkness but directs us toward the emergence of a familiar comforting light. That Grey's performance is a cover of a much-celebrated song from the 1960s – a song that has been performed by everyone from John Lennon to U2 to Tracy Chapman – reflects a return to what is familiar, a reawakening of a treasured past. Because "Stand by Me" is so famous, many viewers will already anticipate the chorus that is not reached in the ad: "So darling, darling, stand by me." For those viewers who already know which words are to come, the chorus starts to play in their head as soon as the ad is over, the music creating the sensation that comfort and familiarity lie just around the corner. Like the experience of driving, the beloved song, lying dormant in the viewer's mind, is ready to wake up.

Skylar Grey's distinctly melancholy version of the song was originally recorded for the Budweiser Super Bowl commercial "Stand by You,"[30] which aired in 2018. This ad, filmed in response to recent natural disasters such as Hurricane Harvey, which had devastated Houston in 2017, shows Budweiser employees rearranging the brewery production line to fill cans with water, rather than beer, for distribution in disaster-struck regions, an act of goodwill that Budweiser has performed many times in the past. The message of "Stand by You" – that acts of solidarity and perseverance will allow for recovery after a disaster – is thus echoed by the use of the same recording in "Sleeping Roads." The message from Mazda is that Covid is one of many natural disasters we have collectively endured and that society will recover from the pandemic just as it has recovered from the fires and floods of the past.[31]

A few weeks after the airing of "Sleeping Roads," as the initial lockdown restrictions were just starting to be lifted in Canada and the United States near the end of May, Mazda produced a new version of the ad. In this version, Grey sings the chorus that had been withheld in the original ad, and the tagline is replaced with a new message: "Together we can take on the road ahead."[32] The roads, this ad tells us, are just beginning to wake up, and it's time for us to start driving again (a sentiment that turned out to be rather premature, given the recurring virus waves and lockdowns yet to come). Although comments about awakening "into a new world" can use the image of sleep to embrace a sense of radical change, the Mazda ads use sleep as a soothing figure for a cyclical return to the habitual. At stake in these contrasting deployments of sleep is the question of whether the pandemic should be seen as an interlude – a mere interruption of the status quo of consumer capitalism – or as the onset of a cultural transformation in which the habits and ideologies of the past can no longer be assumed.

Here, we can return once again to Simon J. Williams's argument in *The Politics of Sleep* that current discourse about sleep can be categorized as belonging to either the "sleep-negative agenda," the "sleep-positive agenda," or the "critical-reflexive agendas."[33] "Sleeping Roads" seems to complicate Williams's theory. The ad cannot really be called sleep-positive (as it does not promote actual sleep), it is not a critical-reflexive text that investigates the politics of sleep, and it is not necessarily sleep-negative. Yes, the ad looks forward to when the roads will wake, but it would be reductive to say that the ad invalidates sleep or portrays sleep as an affront. Rather, the ad seems to respect the need for dormancy, allowing us to linger in the eerily beautiful silent world as we "let the roads sleep." The key to the way that this ad confounds Williams's theory is that the ad both is and is not about sleep at all. It embraces the figure of sleep but uses it for other purposes altogether. Perhaps, to Williams's matrix, we can add a fourth category – "figurative agendas" – to account for representations that use the image or notion of sleep to enforce particular values, a process that does not necessarily neglect or invalidate sleep but builds meaning through visions of sleep as a symbolic figure.

This notion of the figurative agenda is also in line with Cressida Heyes's assertion that "representations of sleep are increasingly deployed within existing scripts of class, race, and gender stratification."[34] (You may recall Heyes's example of "Sleeping Beauty," where Little Briar Rose falls asleep and passively waits, without agency, for the male prince to arrive.) We might usefully see "Sleeping Roads" and other such texts from a similar point of view. In the car ad, sleep is deployed to reinforce automobile culture, which is to say not only that the ad plays to class values around mobility but also that it resists any action that would threaten the "existing script" of consumer culture and carbon emissions.

Representations of sleep during the lockdowns thus contributed to larger conversations about whether the pandemic could or should enable long-term radical cultural changes. In 2020, science fiction author Kim Stanley Robinson observed (perhaps optimistically) that the pandemic had prompted society to attach a new sense of value to things that had often been taken for granted, such as food, health care, and education, as well as to the people who provide these necessities. "The virus," he declared, "is rewriting our imaginations. What felt impossible has become thinkable ... We seem to be learning our way into a new structure of feeling."[35] Although Robinson didn't include it in his list, sleep is surely among those undervalued elements of daily life that deserve renewed attention and that could benefit from a new structure of feeling. Creating a new imaginative structure of sleep will require attention not just to the literal practice of sleeping but also to the figurative representations through which sleep gives shape to expressions of hope, nostalgia, and loss. Contested visions of sleep can reflect unequal approaches to actual slumber, but they can also constitute a proxy war between opposing sides of far-reaching cultural issues. Sleep is a reflection of values, and a literacy of sleep can cast light on what kind of world we want to wake up to after a period of disruptive change.

4

Entering Sleep Mode

THE MOST FREQUENT everyday encounter with a cultural representation of sleep, for many people, is the sleep/wake function on their phones. We place our phones and computers into sleep mode when we finish using them, and then we wake them up again, often just a few seconds later, when we feel an urge to check the weather or send a message, a process that often repeats around a hundred times a day.[1] Sleep mode implies that the purpose of sleep is to enter a state of readiness, as the device (like its user) is always on the verge of the next opportunity to embrace productivity or entertainment. Meanwhile, the distinction between sleep and wakefulness is continually blurred by chimes and notifications that pop up even when the phone is otherwise inert on a table. A sleeping phone might wake up at any moment, even when its human user is trying to get in a nap.[2] An irony of the digital age is that ubiquitous devices that come equipped with a sleep button have contributed to widespread sleep loss, especially among young people.[3]

That this representation of sleep is both so uneasy and so ubiquitous reflects the larger role of technologies of sleep as ambivalent forces within our lives, particularly when devices move beyond their own sleep modes and try to optimize the actual sleep of their human users. Machines, trackers, and apps can illuminate the nature of sleep even as they alter it in ways both subtle and overt. They can usher us dreamily into an algorithmically measured world of restful slumber even while they amplify our insomniac anxieties. Technology tends to be understood, paradoxically, as both the source of disrupted sleep and its potential remedy, a conundrum that has existed for many years. Benjamin Reiss points out that in the nineteenth century, "trains and telegraphs were also said to produce a frantic pace in people's lives that led to unnatural sleep. Then as now, novel technology was thought to be both the cause of and cure for insomnia ... Victorians deployed all manner of electrified sleep gadgetry, including belts, rods, brushes, and even a vibrating helmet to induce the sleep that seemed so difficult to attain in their frantic, hyperconnected world."[4] Indeed, Michael Greaney observes that sleep has always been "an event at the interface of the natural and the technological," even though modern devices present radically new capabilities and demand new forms of evaluation.[5] Whereas technological optimists point to today's sleep-tracking gadgets and colour-shifting light bulbs as ushering in a new era of optimized slumber, skeptics wonder how the same technologies that keep our brains wired into continuous hits of dopamine could possibly be repackaged as real sleep aids.

Earlier in this book, I examined sleep products by looking at mattress ads, if not so much at the actual mattresses. Here, I look more closely at what it means to live with technologies of sleep, particularly through the ambivalence of digital technologies, and I suggest that if we want to understand the products that shape our sleep, we need to engage closely with matters of narrative. The way that we interact with technologies of sleep is a combined function of the design of the objects themselves and the narratives through which these objects reflect particular values. Although consumer technologies might seem to pull people's attention away from the more contemplative acts of reading associated with novels and poems, the ability to identify and assess narratives remains as vital as ever. The narratives built into technologies of sleep have the ability to shape what sleep means, both for sleepers and for those who are kept awake.

Matthew Walker, the director of UC Berkeley's Center for Human Sleep Science and the author of *Why We Sleep*, is among the optimists, arguing that instead of fighting technology, we should embrace it. His book presents a long list of reasons that sleep-tracking features in apps, phones, cars, and homes will help us to improve our sleep quality by setting up personalized sleep zones of light, temperature, and bedtime scheduling.[6] These technologies will give us personalized data about our sleep, correlated with carefully tracked records of our personal work productivity and mood changes, which we can then act on to improve our sleep and our lives. For instance, an app could help someone reduce their likelihood of developing Alzheimer's disease by adjusting their sleep habits, which in turn could contribute to a "sleep credit" score that could be used to lower their health insurance rates.[7] Individuals will have the tools that they need to assess their own sleep, and their smart devices, like loving parents, will dim the lights and close the curtains at just the right time in the evening.

Although Walker enjoys the utopian promise of this imagined future, one can also envision a scenario in which sleep-tracking technologies bring about a dystopian world of terrifying surveillance and patronizing control. Imagine, for instance, that you arrive home late from work after struggling through a busy day. As you scramble to make a late dinner, the light bulbs in your house dim to a red hue to encourage melatonin production. Squinting through the feeble light, you serve the dinner, clean the kitchen, make the kids' lunches for the next day, and tell the kids to clean up their toys. Your phone rings; it's your elderly parent, who needs your help to get to a medical appointment tomorrow. Meanwhile, Alexa, your friendly digital assistant, activates a smart speaker in your kitchen and says, "To get the best sleep, now would be a great time to get ready for bed." You dismiss Alexa. You make the kids a bedtime snack, clean up their toys, negotiate with them about brushing their teeth, get them into bed, and read them a story. Once they drift off, you get up and check your work email; a minor crisis has arisen, and you need to send a few messages. The hour grows late, but you are too wound up to go to bed, and this is also your only chance to enjoy some time to yourself, so you watch some television, and then toss and turn under the covers before finally entering a restless slumber. In the morning, you wake up to a friendly voice. "Good morning," Alexa says. "You did not get sufficient sleep last night. Your risk of a heart attack and early death has increased by 1 per cent. Your health insurance premium has increased by thirty-five cents. It looks like you'll need some help staying awake today. I've just placed an order for more of your favourite coffee beans. During your insufficient sleep, it looks like you had a dream about your ex. I've selected a sad songs playlist. This dream analysis was sponsored by Tinder, which is offering a 20 per cent discount. Would you like to subscribe?"[8]

This dystopian future and the utopian one imagined by Walker are of course essentially the same scenario. The Venn diagram of these two futures would look like a single circle. (In fairness, Walker does not recommend caffeine, but Amazon certainly would.) A digital assistant peering into one's dreams may sound outlandish, but scientists can already use MRI scans to read the general content of a sleeper's dreams.[9] If some enterprising manufacturer of apps and trackers offered a cheaper alternative, such dream scans could conceivably be accomplished in one's bedroom, with a person's dreams siphoned off each night in the context of corporate surveillance for the purpose of targeted advertising or self-improvement.[10]

The utopian vision, in assuming that any sleep problem must have a technological solution, tends to disregard a number of problems. Technologies that are hyper-individualized, to the point where family members are given different sleep zones in the same house, may improve sleep in certain ways, yet they also reinforce the neoliberal notion that individuals must take personal responsibility for problems that are in fact largely structural. The cultural forces of overwork and stress (so often tied to digital technologies), as well as the realities of caregiving and other commitments, mean that many people will inevitably fail to live up to the solutions provided by the apps and gadgets. What is more, this problem is heavily tied to matters of inequity associated with gender, poverty, and race. People who are time-poor due to structural inequities are more likely to find themselves unable to stick to idealized notions of sleep hygiene, a deficiency for which they could be disproportionately punished under a regime of corporate technological sleep monitoring.

In her article "How Silicon Valley Sets Time," sociologist Judy Wajcman considers the increasingly significant role of digital calendars in daily experiences of time, and her insights are useful for thinking about how technology mediates sleep. Calendar apps, which are ubiquitous on smartphones and computers and can interact in complex ways with other digital assets such as email, maps, and contacts, may seem innocuous. However, Wajcman notes that "calendars increasingly play a fundamental role in establishing our everyday rhythms, shaping our consciousness of temporality."[11] Embedded in the grid of the calendar alongside the deadlines and appointments are cultural assumptions about effective time management, productivity, and the "long-standing but mistaken belief, hegemonic in Silicon Valley, that automation will deliver us more time."[12] Although calendars "can provide a source of positive identity and a sense of accomplishment," they also embody a management function that "routinely sets up personal failure, as lived time rarely matches ideals or intentions."[13] Wajcman draws a parallel to the famous industrial efficiency obsession of the turn of the twentieth century, where management consultant Frederick Taylor used a stopwatch to devise ideal sequences of timed motions for repetitive tasks. But whereas Taylor, at least, didn't follow the factory workers home after their shift, "24/7 mobile connectivity has made these boundaries increasingly porous," with the result that "even leisure time is subject to the principles of optimization."[14] The value judgments underlying digital calendars and assistants, Wajcman says, are thus based on "an instrumental philosophy in which an efficient life is morally equated to a good life."[15]

Now that Taylor's stopwatch is following us into our homes and bedrooms, it is easy to see why the technological management of time through consumer products is expanding rapidly into the management of sleep. A sleep-tracking app or a smart light bulb can shape our consciousness of sleep, altering our sense of how, when, and even why we drift off at night. Technological sleep aids may differ from daytime productivity apps in the sense that attaining good sleep is demonstrably helpful for a person's health, whereas increasing daytime productivity involves murkier value judgments. Nevertheless, there is no universal "perfect" sleep that one might attain, and the embeddedness of sleep-tracking products within the larger system of technological culture and its obsessions with efficiency and consumption raises questions about whose interests are served by the optimization of individuals' sleep. In their study of how sleep trackers reinforce the notion of the "Quantified Self," Diletta De Cristofaro and Simona Chiodo argue that "the drive to self-improve at the heart of self- and sleep-tracking props up an understanding of the self that is centred around achievement. This understanding ends up devaluing sleep and risks contributing to the sleep crisis."[16] The obsessively quantified self, we might say, is unlikely to be a truly restful self. De Cristofaro and Chiodo also note, "In this context, sleep becomes just another achievement to 'unlock,' to draw on the vocabulary of gamification that often characterises self-tracking technologies."[17] Indeed, some of the design techniques used in sleep-tracking apps, which reward the user with high scores, streaks, and trophies, are drawn directly from the principles of addictive mobile phone games. Consumer technology and good sleep can make for strange bedfellows.

Moreover, just as the rigorous use of productivity apps is not necessarily the best way to make "good" use of a person's time, the ability of sleep-assisting technologies to produce good sleep, or any sleep at all, is by no means assured. A gadget-free bedroom is often touted as a key element of good sleep hygiene, yet we are meant to measure and enforce this hygiene by equipping our bedroom with all manner of biometric trackers, smart mattresses, and phone apps. Finally, by recording the timing, quality, and phases of a person's sleep in painstaking detail, tracking devices convey the notion that this data is important and that users must dedicate themselves to controlling what is now being measured, a prospect that is easily at odds with the relaxed state of mind necessary for good sleep. There is a sense in which you can only ever fall asleep by mistake, and if you focus on how much you need sleep, you might not be able to get it. Sleep aid technologies can paradoxically increase our frantic craving for sleep, thus chasing the key moment of accidentally stumbling into dreamland further and further away.

The Pod Pro mattress, created by a company called Eight Sleep, is a typical example. A phone app allows you to warm or cool the Pod Pro to precise temperatures in four scheduled stages throughout the night, creating a worrying new domain of expertise for you to research and strategize. In the morning, the mattress vibrates at chest level to wake you up, and the app then displays immensely complex charts and graphs of your sleep data, including obscure but alarming warnings about your heart rate variability.[18] It is hardly surprising that among sleep researchers whose patients suffer from insomnia due to a desperate fixation on their sleep-tracking data, a new term, "orthosomnia," has been coined to refer to "an unhealthy obsession with achieving perfect sleep."[19] This is not even to speak of what happens when the products go wrong. The temperature settings on the Pod Pro run a surprisingly extreme range from 12.8 to 43.3 degrees Celsius. We might infer from past experience with connected technologies that hackers could almost certainly find a way to ransom unsuspecting Pod Pro users under threat of nonstop freezing or roasting.

Even those devices that seem to embody a more gentle design philosophy often remain ensnared within the problematic context of technological utopianism. The "Night Shift" mode on Apple's iPhones, which is meant to foster healthy circadian rhythms by reducing the screen's blue light wavelengths when the sun sets in your location, was touted as a model of sleep-friendly innovation. However, when researchers ran a controlled experiment to test the feature, they found that "there were no differences in sleep outcomes attributable to Night Shift."[20] One possible factor in this result is that interacting with a phone is not just a matter of exposing your retinas to different colour temperatures but also involves "the psychological engagement experienced when texting, scrolling and posting."[21] Likewise, an iPhone feature called "Sleep Mode" (a phrase that now refers to the state of the user, not just the phone) hides notifications to protect your nighttime hours from distraction, but a companion feature called "Wind Down" brings up suggestions to open various apps that feature "journaling, meditating, listening to music, listening to a Podcast, reading, checking off tasks on the calendar, yoga, and more," creating a seemingly endless to-do list at bedtime.[22] Part of the problem is that the technology industry becomes caught up in its own relentless competitive pressure to build ever more comprehensive sleep-assisting and -tracking features into its products. When Apple added a sleep-tracking feature to the Apple Watch in 2020, the developers focused on an overall picture of sleep duration, consciously avoiding presenting the user with complicated REM graphs because "it can be overwhelming and stressful to look at that data."[23] Two years later, however, Apple joined competitors such as Fitbit in presenting exactly these measurements, showing the user "how much time you spent in REM, core, or deep sleep, as well as when you might have woken up."[24] Do companies launch these features to help people sleep or because they can't let their competitors get ahead? Inherent to technological utopianism is the uneasy but frantic need to sell the most advanced and impressive sleep products possible.

Unlike the users of these products, who may choose to grapple with their contradictions, the people who manufacture the devices, far from benefiting from the sleep-assisting features of the gadgets that they are assembling, may be subjected to severe sleep disruptions. Considering the iPhone 5c model as an example, Reiss notes that the employees who assembled the phones had to work 11.5 hour shifts "with only a thirty-minute meal break." Meanwhile, "day-shift and night-shift workers in the plant were made to sleep eight to a dorm room, stacked on hard, narrow cots, where they suffered inevitable interruptions of sleep as their roommates came and went on different schedules."[25] Several years and several iPhone models later, Bloomberg reporters witnessed nearly identical conditions at another facility, with workers living in humid, musty, overcrowded dorm rooms.[26] A photograph taken at a manufacturing complex shows workers in outdoor coats sleeping in a cafeteria, slumped over at the hard tables, their heads resting on their arms. After the devices have been manufactured and sold, the users who run into problems and call a customer support line may have their calls answered by further sleep-deprived workers, agents on the other side of the world who must stay awake at night to make themselves available during the waking hours of wealthier nations.[27] Jonathan Crary argues that capitalism will inevitably seek to do away with sleep altogether because profits can be maximized through the creation of "the sleepless worker or consumer."[28] Just as troubling, however, is a scenario where only *certain* people are made sleepless to serve the interests of the wealthy few, whose sleep is lovingly orchestrated through heart rate scans and luxury mattresses. For certain definitions of sleepless, this scenario has already occurred.

In 2021, the sleep aid industry was valued at over US$64 billion,[29] and even though consumer sleep technologies can be useful in many ways, we must be aware of their intense contradictions, the often silent values that they enforce, the inequities built into their supply chains, and their assumptions about the populations to which they cater. The same products that are designed to foster and protect good sleep may in fact reveal how the notion of the sleep-positive agenda is often predicated on conditions that are hostile to restful recuperation. Indeed, Simon J. Williams sees the sleep-negative agenda as characterized by the individualization, privatization, and depoliticization of sleep, all of which tend to characterize consumer sleep technologies.[30]

A curious compatibility is thus visible in the way that technologies for enhancing sleep, insofar as they can create painful sleep anxieties, share certain characteristics with technologies for preventing sleep. Consider, for example, the notion of "defensive design," a strategy adopted in cities across Canada and elsewhere that aims to prevent loitering and crime by making sleep impossible in public spaces.[31] Defensive design takes the form of a third armrest in the middle of a park bench. It takes the form of carefully spaced planters along walls, metal studs on platforms, and boulders and spikes embedded in the ground, all carefully installed to prevent public sleeping (as well as other illicit activities such as skateboarding). City space is shared space, and the tensions visible in defensive design can reflect legitimate competing needs. Bright lighting and surveillance cameras, for instance, can be important for discouraging assault, especially against women, yet secluded places free of garish illumination and aggressive scrutiny can be vital refuges for those who are homeless. If sleep is a fundamental human need, and public space in the city is increasingly a sleep-free zone, what happens to people without a private place to spend their nights? A bench with a third armrest is not unlike the "Wind Down" feature; it promotes relaxation while making true rest very difficult.

Social housing advocates have observed that people without homes are initially punished through the absence of adequate housing and shelters and again punished for needing an outdoor place to sleep.[32] Under these circumstances, even though defensive design is clearly a sleep-negative approach for those targeted, we cannot simply respond to the issue by declaring war on mid-bench armrests. Focusing narrowly on the importance of sleep in this case would sidestep the larger issue: defensive design to prevent public sleeping is a symptom of society's failure to address inequality and homelessness. The problem arises not from an undervaluing of sleep per se but from an undervaluing of social equity and justice. This is one sense in which we must be cautious about categorizing social practices as either sleep-negative or sleep-positive. Defensive design, as an attack on sleep, comes about not just as a matter of installing anti-sleep objects but also as a byproduct of other forms of value to do with who is excluded from the dominant public sphere. If somebody can't sleep, they may indeed need a better bed and pillows, but we shouldn't just equip them with new sleep technologies and walk away; we should confront the structural forces that may have excluded them from good slumber in the first place.

In critiquing technologies of sleep, we must take care not to make the erroneous claim that technology-free sleep is beneficial, or even possible. As I mentioned in chapter 1, a mattress is not a ruse or a fad – and vital technologies of sleep can also include blankets, shelter, and in a rapidly warming world, air conditioning. Within the context of sleep health care and sleep science research (domains that most people do not encounter as often as they do consumer products), technologies such as sleep apnea masks and EEGs have opened many rich possibilities for improving our understanding of sleep and, for some people, the actual quality of sleep. Sleep science labs, with their wires, cameras, charts, and graphs, have tended to be viewed with deep suspicion by writers of fiction and memoir, yet these labs can provide crucial diagnoses, and the treatments offered in sleep clinics can at times be life-changing. Anthropologist Matthew Wolf-Meyer argues that sleep clinics can uphold inspiring standards of bioethics and that it would be a mistake to see the sleep clinic "as solely the site of disciplining and controlling bodies."[33] Likewise, the sleep technologies that make their way into our bedrooms can inspire creative and useful approaches to sleep even as they raise well-founded misgivings. Greaney asserts that due to ubiquitous sleep trackers, "soon all bedrooms will be sleep labs, if we so wish, and the sleep lab will become a thing of the past."[34] We will need to decide, each night, who and what our bedroom sleep labs are for. Which sleep interventions are empowering, and which ones are manipulative? When is it okay for others to benefit from our REM cycles? Which decisions should fall to individuals, and which ones require regulation and oversight? The answer is not to somehow reject technology or scientific curiosity but to develop a critical literacy of sleep objects (and the discourse surrounding them) that accounts for our messy encounters with complex products and representations. Somewhere at the intersection of the utopian and dystopian visions of sleep technology is a complex and shifting set of consequences that we must learn to negotiate alongside all the other forces in our lives. By way of a case study in this negotiation, let's take a peek into the world of Calm, the home of Sleep Stories.

SLEEP STORIES

Calm is a smartphone app that bills itself as "The #1 app for Sleep, Meditation and Relaxation."[35] Sold through an annual subscription, the app features recorded guided meditations, relaxing music, and tutorials on topics such as "Stoic Wisdom for Modern Life" and "Radical Self-Compassion."[36] Created in 2012 by Michael Acton Smith and Alex Tew, and based in San Francisco, Calm was named Apple's "App of the Year" in 2017. By 2019, having famously secured venture funding from Ashton Kutcher, Calm was the top-grossing iPhone health and fitness app and was valued at US$1 billion.[37] In 2020, Calm partnered with HBO to launch a television series called *A World of Calm*, comprised of dreamy, sleep-inducing nature documentaries narrated by Lucy Liu, Nicole Kidman, Keanu Reeves, and Idris Elba, among others.[38] Like so many products that emphasize self-care in a stressed-out world, Calm has tapped into a big, thirsty market.

The obvious difficulties that apply to many sleep-based consumer products arise very quickly when considering the Calm media empire. Sleeplessness and anxiety, this kind of product implies, are problems to be solved by individuals, who must choose the best meditation app, pay the hefty subscription fee ($76.99 annually at time of writing),[39] and use the guided meditations with diligence. This approach can be appealing to many users, yet it presents a troubling, neoliberal vision of a world where peace of mind is stockpiled behind a paywall. Even for those who can afford it, the idea of resisting the stresses of modern life with the help of the glitzy, high-tech, celebrity-fuelled mentality of Silicon Valley seems amusingly problematic. As journalist Carrie Battan observes in the *New Yorker*, "There is, of course, a deep contradiction running through phrases such as 'star-studded meditation content' or 'venture-funded meditation service.'"[40] Smartphone apps, more than any other product category on earth, tend to be uniquely blamed for driving the epidemics of stress, distraction, and sleeplessness plaguing modern society. The idea of a phone app to foster meditation and rest sounds almost satirical.

Still, these apps cannot be written off too hastily. Calm has over 100 million downloads and in 2018 was named by the nonprofit Center for Humane Technology as the "'world's happiest app' – the single app that left users feeling happiest from spending time on it, based on data collected from a pool of 200,000 iPhone users."[41] There must be something to this appraisal. And, given my own interest in sleep and narrative, I find myself particularly intrigued by a feature in the Calm app known as Sleep Stories. Essentially serving as bedtime stories for adults, Sleep Stories are slow, meandering narratives in audio form, read aloud by celebrity performers. As Smith puts it, "You've heard of slow food and slow cinema. Now meet slow literature – half literature, half sleep, and totally relaxing."[42] Calm is not alone in offering this kind of feature – the *New York Times* has observed that "the adult bedtime story industry is booming"[43] – but the app is certainly among the best known and most widely used. Calm has a team of Sleep Story authors, all of whom work diligently to break the standard rules of narrative entertainment; a Sleep Story must have almost no conflict or tension, and it must provide no real reason for the listener to reach the ending. If a Sleep Story works, the listener will never hear it all the way through.

The head of Sleep Stories at Calm, and a Sleep Story author himself, is Chris Advansun, a former marketing executive for tech and advertising companies who lives in Toronto. Also trained as a screenwriter, Advansun notes in a Calm blog post, "In film, stories must contain certain elements to hook audience attention and deliver an emotionally satisfying experience: things like desire, obstacles, conflict, tension, and complications. Sleep Stories are different. They are narrative, but instead of building up tension and stakes, the idea is to unwind."[44] In an interview with the CBC, Advansun elaborates on the subtle sense of balance in Sleep Stories, in that the story should very gently "hook the attention of the listener," even though "the goal is for the listener to not get to the end."[45] The story won't work if the listener starts thinking about other things, but it must also seek to extinguish the very attention that it holds, sending the listener into the oblivion of sleep.

You've probably never heard of Chris Advansun. His name does not appear on bestseller lists, on undergraduate literary studies syllabuses, or in the Canada Reads literary competition, but whereas some of the most successful authors in Canada would be lucky to reach 100,000 readers, Advansun's Sleep Stories have been downloaded millions of times,[46] making him, by that measure, one of the most popular Canadian fiction writers of all time. In the Calm app, Advansun's Sleep Stories are read by celebrities with immense pop culture reach, such as Matthew McConaughey and LeVar Burton. If literary scholars want to meet the public where their attention lies, we need to be paying attention to Sleep Stories.

In the interest of research, then, I decided one summer to embrace mindfulness and give Calm a try. Accessing the service through the app's website, amusingly named Calm.com, I completed part of the registration process only to discover that Calm has no weekly, monthly, or one-time purchase options – only the steep annual fee of $76.99. I decided to think it over a little before entering my credit card number, so I closed the site and went about my day. Over the next fifteen hours, one email after another from Calm popped up in my inbox. "Don't forget to breathe," advised one email, showing an animated guided-breathing icon. "Paul, your discount is inside," said another message. The next email came from "Christi from Calm," who informed me that she was "following up on our offer." All these emails from Calm were stressing me out! And they didn't stop: "Better sleep can start tonight," said the next one. And then: "Paul, take just 10 minutes for your mental fitness." At this point, as much to make the emails stop as anything, I subscribed to the seven-day free trial and installed Calm on my phone. Immediately, the app asked permission to send me push notifications and to view my activity across other apps. These functions, I could not help thinking, did not bode well for mindfulness and relaxation.

In any case, I now had access to the Sleep Stories. Most of the Sleep Stories are original fiction, although the app also includes selections from works in the public domain, such as *Anne of Green Gables*, *The Wind in the Willows*, and (sorry, old-school English professors) Shakespeare's sonnets. The names of the hired Sleep Story authors are buried in small print behind the marquee display showing the celebrity performer, but because of my interest in Canadian writers, I tracked down Advansun's stories, which include "Wonder" ("a dreamy story about the mysteries of the universe" performed by Matthew McConaughey), "Journey to the Stars" ("an awe-inspiring journey across our beloved solar system" with LeVar Burton), "Song of the Sunbird" (a "moonlight quest through the jungles of Kilimanjaro" with Leona Lewis), and several others.[47]

I settle on a story called "The Butterfly Sanctuary," performed by Clarke Peters, an actor from *The Wire* and *John Wick*,[48] who, Calm notes, is "world renowned for his mellifluous voice." This is a daytime listening session for me, so I won't be trying to fall asleep. I just want to see how the story works. I press the play button, and Peters's voice, which truly is wonderful, floats through the air in liquid, soothing tones:

> My name is Clarke Peters, and tonight I'll be reading you a Sleep Story called "The Butterfly Sanctuary." Before we begin, let's take a moment to settle in and relax. Cozy up under the covers and find a comfortable position. Then, when *you're* ready, close your eyes. Become aware of the bed supporting your body. Let your legs and hips and back sink into the mattress. Allow the weight of your head to ease down into the pillow. And to help you embrace the peace and stillness of this moment, let's take a few mindful breaths, inhaling deeply and exhaling slowly.

After some more guided breathing, Peters says, "And with that, let's start today's story." The rhetorical technique here, in which the lengthy preparatory remarks push back the beginning of the story, serves a dual function. First, it establishes a relationship between the storyteller and the listener based on their agreement that the storytelling event is to take place within a specific real-world setting, a bedroom where the teller will be guiding the listener to sleep. This notion of the story as an event, an idea that tends to be associated with oral storytelling traditions, is largely foreign to most works of written or filmed fiction, which make no explicit presumptions as to the actual situation of the reader or viewer. The Sleep Story, then, is situated within the oral tradition but also belongs to the transactional model of literature, much loved in the children's publishing industry, that is embodied by bedtime stories whose purpose is to put the kid to sleep. The Sleep Story gives adult listeners permission to release themselves from responsibility, to be held in the arms (or the mellifluous voice) of a trusted figure who will make everything seem alright. The oral tradition and the children's bedtime genre are both fairly unusual in being applied so overtly to the smartphone-bearing adult citizens of the modern Western world. With one foot in each of these genres, the Sleep Story may have a special appeal, but its effectiveness depends almost entirely on the willingness of the listener not just to listen to the story but also to participate in the storytelling event.

The second function of the prefatory material about cozying up under the covers is that, even though it seems to defer the beginning of the story, it can usefully be understood as *part* of the Sleep Story. These remarks contribute to the tale's narrative function of relaxing listeners and moving them toward sleep. One of the odd things about the lingo of Sleep Stories and ebooks is that the performers who read the stories are known as "narrators," a peculiar use of terminology that tends to ruffle the feathers of literary scholars for whom the narrator of a story is a character, often nameless, whose recounting of events constitutes the story. I would never get away with calling myself the narrator of *Moby-Dick* just because I read the book out loud. In a sense, Peters is no more the narrator of "The Butterfly Sanctuary" than I am of *Pride and Prejudice*; the story is told in free indirect discourse from a third-person point of view, the narrator rendered as a nameless fictional figure invested in the experiences of the central character. Yet, in "The Butterfly Sanctuary," the blurring of the two narrators – Peters and the nameless narrator – into one entity almost seems to be a canny acknowledgment of the fact that the frame narrative, in which Peters tells us to relax and get ready for the story, is part of the tale that we are being told.

Once Peters has established the storytelling event through the frame narrative, the story itself follows an evening in the life of the protagonist, Malik, who steps off a city bus and walks along a downtown street with the goal of "boarding a train to the south end of the city, which would take him to campus for an evening class." Immediately after announcing Malik's intention to find his train, however, the narrative gives itself over to slow, dreamy, sensory descriptions of the gentle sights and sounds along the street. Malik observes the faces and voices of the people around him, notices the leaves of the trees that he passes, and realizes that every sound has a purpose. After a while, he pauses before a man sitting on a bench, and he sees something that holds his attention for a long time:

> Just before Malik turned away and walked on, he noticed the most curious thing perched on the man's shoulder: a beautiful butterfly. Her wings beamed with bright pink stripes set on a black canvas, rounding and flowing in an intricate pattern of curves and waves. The stripes were finer at the inside and grew thicker toward the outside, until giving way to a vibrant purple ridge that contoured the wing's edges. The butterfly sat there, so stunning and so still, Malik wondered if she was real. But she moved her wings just a little, as if to reassure passersby that the universe did indeed produce such magical things as this.

This lengthy description, like most of the Sleep Story, strategically defers the plot. Indeed, eight minutes into the story, Malik's catching a train toward campus for an evening class remains the only identifiable plot element, and a notional one at that, since it hasn't yet occurred. The narrative, quite intentionally, is a story only in the loosest possible terms, as Malik's movement through the city serves more as a guided sensory meditation than a driver of events.

The function of the Sleep Story to defer the plot by dedicating close attention to a stream of sensory elements bears a surprising resemblance to the techniques of literary fiction, in which plot is often de-emphasized in favour of the development of imagery and explorations of interiority. Malik's journey to campus for his evening class is not unlike Mrs Dalloway's journey to buy the flowers; the famous first sentence of Virginia Woolf's novel – "Mrs. Dalloway said she would buy the flowers herself"[49] – establishes a seemingly central act that is, in a vital sense, of no importance whatsoever. Important is the exploration of consciousness that occurs along the way. In "The Butterfly Sanctuary," Malik finally turns away from the captivating butterfly and, almost as though in homage to *Mrs. Dalloway*, walks by a flower shop and takes "a deep, satisfying breath, delighting in the scent of the orchids and roses and lilacs." Yet, whereas Woolf's fiction is invested in untangling the experience of consciousness through a deeply developed representation of subjectivity, "The Butterfly Sanctuary" tells us very little about Malik. He remains nearly featureless, serving as a vehicle for listeners to direct their imaginative attention toward mildly absorbing sensations. Another genre to which the Sleep Story bears a striking resemblance is the shaggy dog story, a meandering tale whose purpose is not to lead to a narrative destination but to see how long it can string the listener along for no reason. A Sleep Story eschews the centrality of plot like literary fiction, and it takes form through long-winded digressions like a shaggy dog story, but it skilfully rejects the payoffs of both genres – deep knowledge of subjectivity, on the one hand, and maddening humour, on the other – developing a distinct genre focused on guided sensorial focus.

"The Butterfly Sanctuary" runs in this vein for thirty-five minutes. Malik finally boards the train, the butterfly following along beside him, but he loses interest in his destination, and the two companions eventually wander into a park where they cross a bridge to a wondrous sanctuary holding countless butterflies. The original butterfly leads Malik to a hammock filled with blankets and pillows, into which he gratefully sinks. The hammock, Peters tells us in the end, "enfolded his body like a cocoon ... And in moments he dozed off to the deepest, most peaceful sleep he ever had." Malik never does make it to his evening class, and with any luck, the listener will never make it to the end of the story.

In his interview with the CBC, Advansun notes that "in many of the stories, the resolution of the story is that in the end the character falls asleep. That is the ending."[50] This is one of the obvious features that the Sleep Story shares with children's stories of the *Goodnight Moon* variety. Indeed, much of the work that "The Butterfly Sanctuary" does in terms of imagery, setting, and metaphor pushes with varying degrees of subtlety in this direction. The weight of Malik's knapsack, which "hung from both shoulders," forms a psychological tug downward in the direction of sleep. The swaying of the train from side to side creates a rocking motion like a cradle. When Malik's butterfly leads him toward the sanctuary, it floats through a carved wooden archway, a passage through which Malik must proceed, figuratively reflecting the transition into sleep. Whereas *Mrs. Dalloway* builds an understanding of interiority, "The Butterfly Sanctuary" moves listeners into the actual interiority of their own slumber.

A literary analysis of a Sleep Story can help us to understand how it serves as a kind of sleep contract between the listener and the teller. Yet a traditional scholarly analysis can't quite do the job of seeing how the story *works.* Approaching a Sleep Story through the study of narrative form and the lens of close reading will never grant us the final word on how the story behaves within its home ecosystem, as it were. To meet Sleep Stories where they live, I knew that I would have to get to know them on more intimate terms. I would need to invite them into my bedroom.

I have suffered from periodic insomnia for as long as I can remember. Even during group sleepovers as a child, I would lie awake in the dark while, one by one, my friends fell asleep, their gentle snores washing over me, until I was the only one barred from entry into the sleeping world. As an adult, I have continued to be a dedicated practitioner of sleep-onset insomnia (the inability to fall asleep at the beginning of the night), and lately I've also been dabbling impressively in sleep-maintenance insomnia (the inability to fall back to sleep after waking during the night). This history makes me a prime audience, and a tough customer, for Sleep Stories. Even with my new Calm membership in hand, I was not at all confident that the best way to fall asleep would be to bring a smartphone to my bedside table in clear violation of all sensible sleep-hygiene advice, and I was not optimistic that I would be able to nod off with a narrator talking to me, no matter how deferred the plot. As a long-suffering insomniac, however, I was willing to give Sleep Stories a fair try in sending me to dreamland.

Advansun's story "The Ocean Moon," read by Laura Dern, was the Sleep Story to which I decided to fall asleep. "Drift away to the gorgeous voice of Laura Dern," the app advised me, "in this soothing tale of rolling trains, cresting waves, and a quest to the edge of the sea." That didn't sound so bad. However, on top of my suspicions about the wisdom of bringing a phone to bed, I immediately ran into another complication. Because I share a bed with my wife, Niki, I would be able to play the Sleep Story only if we both agreed that we wanted to listen to it. I had quickly dismissed the absurd idea of trying to fall asleep with headphones strapped onto my head or earbuds stuffed into my ears. No, the phone would rest on my nightstand, playing the story through its speaker, filling the bedroom with Laura Dern's gorgeous voice.

When I asked Niki what she thought about the Sleep Story idea, she said, "I'll probably fall asleep pretty quickly. But once I'm sleeping, I get woken up by small noises, so if the story keeps going for very long, it will just wake me up again." "The Ocean Moon" has a runtime of thirty-four minutes, which Niki felt was too long, so we agreed that I would skip ahead just past the halfway point and listen to the final fifteen minutes. This was a painful compromise for me, partly because falling asleep within fifteen minutes would require a heavenly intervention that even Laura Dern might not be able to provide and also because by missing the first half of the story, I wouldn't know what plot elements the narrative would be working so hard to ignore.

Bypassing the first half of the story might seem like a violation of the spirit of the Calm app experience. Compressing a Sleep Story into a rushed time frame is clearly a ridiculous notion, like trying to skip ahead to the end of a meditation session in order to get a sneak peek at what mindfulness feels like. Skipping half of the Sleep Story might make me a good citizen of the acceleration society, but I knew that it wouldn't be fair to Advansun, to Dern, or to myself. Yet the practicalities of listening to the Sleep Story cannot be disentangled from its function as a sleep aid. The listener is supposed to play the Sleep Story when falling asleep, but many listeners share a bedroom with a partner, a baby, or even a group of roommates. These realities cannot suddenly be ignored just because the listener has paid $76.99 for a subscription to a mindfulness app. By presuming to insert itself into my actual life, the Calm app does not enter a vacuum where it can lay claim to my full and undivided being. It enters a messy, complicated family life of shared spaces and consideration for others. My compromise with Niki, then, reflects a very real encounter between a phone meditation app and the experiences of actual people.

And so I drag the location slider for "The Ocean Moon" past the halfway point, find a comfortable spot on my pillow, and try to figure out what Dern is talking about. Sure enough, plot elements are few and far between, as Dern focuses her soothing murmur on the sensory details of a train entering a tunnel and then on a view of a gently pulsing ocean. I worry that the story is a little loud for Niki, so I reach over and lower the volume. Now, I have to strain to hear, so I raise the volume just a little and continue to listen. Although I've never thought about it before, Dern's voice has been familiar to me for most of my life. Her most famous role, which she has been occasionally reprising over an impressive span of thirty years, is that of paleobotanist

Dr Ellie Sattler in the *Jurassic Park* movies.[51] I'll never forget Ellie's astonished face, gaping up from the park jeep, when she sees a brachiosaurus for the first time or her conversation about chaos theory with Ian Malcolm (Jeff Goldblum) while they roll past the tyrannosaur paddock. "Man destroys God. Man creates dinosaurs," says Ian. "Dinosaurs eat man. Woman inherits the earth," Ellie replies.

This famous line about woman inheriting the earth is supposed to land a feminist punch, but as a young viewer, I never noticed the awful, casual misogyny in the movie. When he sees the brachiosaurus before she does, Alan Grant (Sam Neill) grabs the top of Ellie's head and, ignoring the comment that she is making about a resurrected extinct veriforman, forcefully rotates her skull toward the dinosaur until her head reaches an angle that could painfully strain her neck. Ian's explanation of chaos theory, meanwhile, is stunningly patronizing. "Was I going too fast?" he says, with a laugh, while reaching forward, uninvited, and fondling Ellie's blond hair. Even though she has been summoned to the island for her expertise, no one really cares when Dr Sattler identifies toxic plants in the visitor centre or when she notices, much to the surprise of the actual dinosaur veterinarian who is supposed to be treating the sick triceratops, that the animal's pupils are dilated and that it's suffering from Melia toxicity from West Indian lilacs. Everyone in the movie has to try to survive the dinosaurs, but Ellie also has to survive the men. Like so many movies, *Jurassic Park* can be read as a celebration of misogyny – a victory of the men with guns over the all-female dinosaurs – or if you squint just right, as an exposé and critique of the patriarchy. Critic Kayleigh Dray points out that in a 1990s cinematic world of princesses and singing nuns, Ellie was a revolutionary figure, a feminist icon with hiking boots, heroic bloodstains, and a PhD.[52] Niki was a big Ellie Sattler fan as a teenager. I haven't mentioned to her that the voice we are hearing in our Sleep Story is Dern's, and I wonder if she will recognize it. Probably not, since Dern's vocal performance in "The Ocean Moon" is much lower and dreamier than when she plays Ellie. Niki is tossing and turning a little bit. The Sleep Story might be keeping her awake. Wait, what's happening in "The Ocean Moon"? Is Dern still describing the water? I haven't been paying attention! Clearly, when it comes to mindfulness, I am a terrible Sleep Story listener.

Eventually, Dern reaches the uneventful conclusion of the story. As is typical for me, I'm still fully awake. Uncharacteristically, Niki is awake, too. She will tell me the next day that she couldn't sleep with the Sleep Story playing. Advansun's hope is that his audience will only ever hear the first half of "The Ocean Moon," but as fully incompetent Sleep Story listeners, Niki and I have only heard the second half. With no judgment about anyone else's preferences, we seem to find that our marriage is already full enough without inviting Chris Advansun and Laura Dern into the bedroom with us. Only our little daughter Holly, whose bed rests alongside ours, is blissfully unaware that the Sleep Story experiment ever took place.

My distracted thoughts about *Jurassic Park* represent not only a practical difficulty with Sleep Stories but also a political one. The ambition of a Sleep Story is to invite the listener into a dreamy world free of the machinations of oppression and power. However, Dern's connection to problematic Hollywood action flicks is just one example of how Sleep Stories, as with all forms of representation, remain inevitably tied to the preoccupations of waking life. Like a velociraptor in the cafeteria kitchen, the monster of cultural politics tiptoes menacingly through "The Ocean Moon."

Silicon Valley has a well-known diversity problem, with white and Asian men dominating the payroll at Apple, Facebook, Google, and the like.[53] Calm, founded next door to these companies in San Francisco by two white men, has been in the similarly precarious position of insinuating their products, which may be developed with limited representation from diverse backgrounds and worldviews, into the most intimate moments of the lives of millions of people. During Calm's rise to a billion-dollar company, the Sleep Story writers included women such as Julie Aigner-Clark (the founder of the Baby Einstein Company, which produces multimedia products for babies), but most of the writers tended to be white Americans, with occasional representation from people of colour such as Wajahat Ali, an American of Pakistani descent.

The Sleep Stories have allowed more diversity among the "narrators," who include Chiké Okonkwo, Bhavnisha Parmar, Fajer Al-Kaisi, Tabitha Brown, and others. However, this partial inclusion tends to lead to a situation, all too prevalent in the entertainment industry, where even though people of colour may gradually be gaining representational ground on-screen, they are still frequently performing stories that are predominantly written by white writers and arranged by white directors and producers. We see this outcome with the Calm app when Black actor Clarke Peters reads Advansun's "The Butterfly Sanctuary" or when Black actor LeVar Burton reads Advansun's

"Journey to the Stars." How should we approach a story like "The Taurus Express," which invites us to "[t]ake a trip from Istanbul to Cairo aboard a historic, luxury train," in light of its performance by Ramon Tikaram, a British actor of Fijian and Southeast Asian descent, and its authorship by the white British novelist Andrew Martin? The cultural and racial implications of such a story might not be especially troublesome if the tale were placed alongside a larger variety of stories written by authors from, say, Turkey and Egypt, but the whiteness of the Sleep Story writers' room raises uncomfortable questions about whose vision of Istanbul – and whose vision of sleep – is presented to the world.

In the wake of the massive Black Lives Matter protests of 2020, Calm was one of many organizations that redoubled their efforts to increase the diversity of representation in their ranks. In early 2021, the Calm blog featured a series of posts called "Meet the Writer behind the Sleep Story," highlighting Black writers.[54] Still, a group photo of Calm's employees, displayed on its website in the same year, showed thirty-four smiling people clustered outdoors, of whom perhaps five appeared to be people of colour, and only one of whom appeared to be Black.[55] This is not to say that their efforts are necessarily insincere but that the problem requires sustained attention. Although Sleep Stories may hope to present sleep as a universal site of release and restoration, visions of sleep always emerge from particular, often inequitable contexts, just as the imagery and plot elements presented in the stories themselves inevitably have connections to sometimes troubling realities. The first episode of the HBO series *A World of Calm*, called "The Coral City," takes place within the coral reef of the Raja Ampat archipelago in Indonesia. The episode presents the reef as a portal into mindfulness and peace, but is it really possible to divorce a coral reef from the crisis of global heating and the acidification of the seas? A Sleep Story asks you to let go of the complexities of oppression, representation, and ecological harm – and letting go of these things is indeed a valuable skill to have late at night – but different writers and listeners cannot all approach this problem on equal ground.

As with other forms of meditation and rest, the participant's position (both literal and figurative) is key. Some listeners will take part in a Sleep Story event much more graciously than I was able to, but the dream-world content of the Sleep Stories can never be fully separated from the cultural politics of the waking world, and the form of the stories as streamable

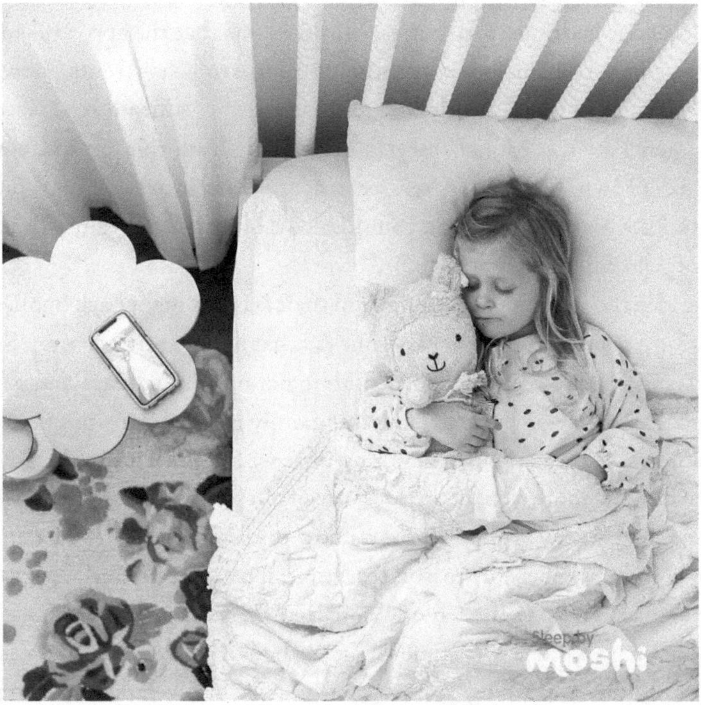

4.1 Mind Candy Ltd Moshi, "Sleep by Moshi," 2020.

content within a phone app cannot easily be disentangled from the sense of perpetual restlessness that digital media tend to inspire. Calm advertises its services as promoting "everyday resilience," but as we have seen, the notion of resilience tends to take a combative stance toward the world, a stance that requires fuelling up individuals each night so that they can bounce back into relentless productivity.

The situation can be even more troubling when children are involved. A sleep app called Moshi, which operates in partnership with Calm and bills itself as "the #1 sleep app for kids," plays recordings of bedtime stories for children, with "narrators" including Goldie Hawn and Patrick Stewart. All the parent has to do is use the voice command, "Alexa – Please get my kid to sleep," and Moshi takes over, thus "gifting parents with more time to enjoy their evenings."[56] Moshi's ads typically show a parent (or a disembodied hand) pointing a phone, like a magic wand, toward a sleeping child. In some ads the parent is absent altogether, the phone on the nightstand having completely taken over the bedtime story duties. Moshi claims that the app "is used after the traditional bedtime book," yet their promise to give parents "more time to enjoy their evenings" clearly implies that the app is meant to replace, not supplement, the traditional storytime. Drawing from this approach, Calm launched its own "Calm Kids" service in 2021, with a nearly identical pitch to parents: "Let Sleep Stories help your kiddos drift off into dreamland and get more of your Sunday night back."[57]

The idea that parents will get more of their Sunday night back implies that parenting is a loss of time, a kind of time tax that needs a refund. Sleep Stories for kids might be said to transport children not only into dreamland but also into a cultural world where outsourcing family relationships to phone apps is an admirable form of efficiency. Now that we have Sleep Stories, we don't need to lose any more time in the presence of our family. The promise of more free time on Sunday night also shows how perilously thin the dividing line can be between supposedly restful storytime apps and tracking apps. Diletta De Cristofaro and Simona Chiodo note that the phenomenon of quantified sleep tracking and the current moral panic about a pervasive sleep crisis tend to be "mutually reinforcing,"[58] and this argument may be applicable to products beyond obvious trackers such as Wi-Fi-connected mattresses. Bedtime story apps may pitch themselves as a relaxing alternative to products that obsessively chart the user's REM cycles, but a storytime app could easily serve as a tracker and evaluator of a family's nightly habits.

Some of us might be tempted to blame parents for the popularity of these apps, but we should remember that such a cynical dismissal would reproduce the individualistic mentality that gives rise to the apps in the first place. After all, time pressure is a powerful social force, even if its consequences tend to feel isolating and personal. As Hartmut Rosa shows in his study of social acceleration, people often experience a compulsion to use time-saving technologies out of a well-justified fear of falling "behind" in a fast-paced world. "Whoever individually refrains from using time-saving techniques," Rosa writes, "pays the price of a partial desynchronization: she cannot stay 'up to date' and loses opportunities."[59] One can easily imagine the parental Moshi subscribers using their freed-up evening time to respond to work emails, pack the kids' lunches, or even "catch up" on the latest streaming television show that everyone else seems to have already watched. Another effect of this conundrum is that time-saving technologies never actually slow the pace of life.

Rosa notes that such technologies change "the *temporal standards* that underlie our actions and plans."[60] This effect leads people to carry out more actions per unit of time, which increases the perceived pace of life even more.

At their most hopeful, Sleep Stories provide a way to use the pervasive nature of technology against itself, carving out a space where technology can use the power of narrative to focus the listener's attention on the present moment and the importance of recuperation. Such a technology, however, also reinforces the idea that there is no escape from the digital world. The very last thing you experience before falling asleep is the sound of a phone app, and the phone or another tracker will also be the thing that wakes you up. Maybe the problem with Sleep Stories is not so much that they don't always work as intended but more importantly that they prevent the onset of sleep from serving as one of the last refuges from the digital technologies that shape so many of our experiences. As my thoughtful colleague Angie Abdou says, "We need silence to find out what we think."[61] Angie lives in the mountains, and she is talking here about wilderness hikes, not cozying up under the covers, but her comment also makes me think that we shouldn't have to abandon our homes to find silence. If we can't disconnect from our devices and embrace the seclusion of our own thoughts when we are falling asleep, what kind of homes have we made for ourselves? What we risk losing, I think, is not necessarily an idealized notion of sleep as a pristine refuge from the hyperconnected world but instead the chance to find in sleep a silent vantage point from which the frenzy of waking life can be put into perspective. Cressida Heyes notes that the magic of sleep is that it "offers an opportunity to continue existing while taking a break from being myself."[62] Deep sleep probably retains this ability regardless of bedtime phone apps, but the hypnagogic borderline, where waking dissolves into slumber, becomes a contested ground when a Sleep Story fills the room.

One of the concerns at stake here is the matter of whether we should approach bedtime apps from the perspective of their cultural implications or from the perspective of individual experience. Much of my argument throughout this book has been that a cultural vision of sleep is vital for reckoning with the seemingly innocent act of slumber as a site of ideology and power, that focusing on the individual can be a kind of neoliberal trick meant to isolate people as units of profit. Something important will surely be lost, however, if we forget that listening to a bedtime story is a deeply personal experience. Insisting on a blanket argument, as it were, for seeing sleep apps on cultural terms would unwittingly cover up the intimacies of drifting to sleep. Bedtime apps can foster genuine pleasures and good sleep for some people, and it would be condescending to suggest that these people are doing something wrong. (I'm probably just jealous.) In questioning so intently whether Silicon Valley really belongs in your bedroom, maybe I'm neglecting to ask if literary theorists do.

Nevertheless, like it or not, technology and culture are always already waiting for us in bed, and crawling under the covers requires coming to terms with these bedfellows in some way. If your best personal sleep involves a celebrity performance, you are certainly in good company. Not only do bedtime apps have millions of users, but people have been using television, radio, and books to fall asleep for years. Some researchers go so far as to recommend a little screen time before bed, as long as it's done in a calming way.[63] De Cristofaro argues that "[i]f we have a 'sleep goal' at all, it should be to learn to value rest on its own terms,"[64] and although she makes this point in order to resist the troubling emphasis on "sleep goals" in tracking apps, there is no reason that valuing rest on its own terms can't involve personal choices about falling asleep to a bedtime story. Bringing the assessment of sleep technologies back to the level of the individual doesn't have to be a neoliberal trick; it can be a way to embrace the intimacy of your own sleep for your own reasons.

The goal, then, shouldn't necessarily be to banish pixels and speakers from the bedroom but to find the sleep that works for you while also building a public sphere that fosters good sleep for others. This process can respect the fact that everyone has different sleep preferences while recognizing that the colonization of hypnagogia by digital media carries a cultural weight. When we fall asleep to a Sleep Story, we can question to what extent we are embracing good slumber and to what extent we are giving ourselves over to the idea that our sleep depends on, and in some sense belongs to, the digital world and its obsession with endless engagement. The distinction between calming media and insomniac media will be different for different people, but one thing we can hold in common if we want to value our sleep as an intrinsic good is the need to examine what it means for sleep to become entwined with digital life. I can't tell you whether you should listen to Sleep Stories, but we do need to foster a literacy of sleep on both personal and cultural levels if we want to assess the technologies that seek to shape the very nature of slumber.

ENTERING THE SLEEPSIDE IN *ASSEMBLING THE MORROW*

Michael Greaney notes that the sleep science lab often appears in recent works of fiction as a dark figure of invasive, mechanistic visions of sleep, a trend that he sees as a reaction to widespread anxieties about a modern technological sleep crisis. Such stories, he says, "represent the latest episode in a long-standing territorial dispute between art and science over the nature of sleep."[65] Embedded within these narratives is "the technophobic assumption that human sleep, in its irrepressible naturalness, is not a state that is ever going to be satisfactorily 'observed, measured, contained' by the new machinic language of slumber."[66] One of the key insights that emerges from Greaney's discussion is that reducing the complexities of sleep to a battle between art and science, or between "natural" sleep and technologically mediated sleep, is a mistake. There never was an ideal past when sleep offered a pristine refuge from the cultural world. Ever since the invention of bedding, or even the invention of sleeping near others, sleep has always taken place within a cultural and technical apparatus. As technological visions of sleep become increasingly complex, we should approach them with curiosity and care as well as a sense of skepticism and critical awareness.

One could easily extend Greaney's observations about novels to nonfiction accounts of sleep labs, such as Christopher Dewdney's description in *Acquainted with the Night* of his one-night stay in the sleep lab at St Michael's Hospital in Toronto. Dewdney's anxiety about the lab is evident in his close attention to the electrodes taped to his calves, temples, scalp, and chin, the equipment attached to his neck, abdomen, finger, and chest, the breathing tube in his nose, and the video camera that watches his every toss and turn.[67] "I was a mass of wires and electrodes," he writes.[68] Unnerved by the fact that the technician reading the brainwave scan knows exactly when he is awake, Dewdney lies in bed unable to sleep for hours, dreading the notion that "they were inside my head."[69] Like many works of narrative fiction, such an account casts suspicion on the techniques of the lab and portrays sleep science as getting in the way of good sleep. Still, Dewdney emerges from the lab with a new piece of knowledge – he suffers from a minor sleep apnea – hinting at how sleep science usefully illuminates certain aspects of sleep, even if the electrodes are unsettling. In reading this narrative, we have the chance to learn from the ambivalence, and even the absurdity, of Dewdney's experience while also questioning whether such an account is fair to the genuine sense of decency and curiosity that motivates sleep scientists.

Greaney's insights, then, have much to offer in considering works of literary fiction and memoir, but as we have seen, poetry can tell another story altogether, operating outside the usual conventions of narrative. In the service of such unexpected possibilities, I close this chapter with a look at a work of experimental poetry that engages with sleep technology. Whereas sleep phone apps advance a transactional use of technology in order to instill sleep and whereas novels use the structures of narrative sequence to build thematic visions of sleep labs and other technologies, a poetics of sleep can experiment more freely with surprising ways of questioning what it means to orient our visions of sleep through a technological lens. Such poetry both honours and resists the dominance of science in encountering sleep, an exercise that provides unique glimpses into what it might mean for us to perceive sleep in its own right.

Swiss Canadian writer Sandra Huber carries out a remarkable poetic investigation of sleep in *Assembling the Morrow: A Poetics of Sleep*. In 2010, Huber held the unusual position of poet in residence at a sleep laboratory at the University of Lausanne in Switzerland.[70] Her goal in this position was to figure out how to represent sleep in language. Such a project immediately encounters the familiar question of how we might be able to perceive the world of sleep – what she calls "the sleepside" – when our notion of perception belongs to waking life. "Part of the reason consciousness remains a mystery," she writes, "is that sleep can't be recognized, and the reason sleep can't be recognized is because we're looking at it while we're wide awake. To meet sleep on its own terms, one should enter not from waking, but from the sleepside. This is an experiment for the moxie of poetics."[71] Because poetry, more than fiction, can release itself from the constraints of narrative and all its fussiness with plot, order, and coherence, poetry is better suited to venturing away from the rationality of waking life.

What, then, would a poetics of sleep look like? In developing an approach to this question, the first half of *Assembling the Morrow* comprises an essay that describes Huber's encounters with the sleep lab as informed by the history of sleep science. Like Dewdney, she emphasizes the contradiction between the intensive surveillance apparatus of the sleep measurement equipment and the need to enter a relaxed sleep. How can normal sleep be studied if the experience of sleeping in a lab is so strange? Nevertheless, Huber insists that the aspiring sleep poet must engage with the sleep lab. Sleep as an object of knowledge, and therefore as an experience, was forever changed by the development of electroencephalographic, or EEG, technology and by the realization that brain activity during sleep could be represented in a chart – *written* as a chaotic line across the page – and categorized into distinct stages of activity. The strangeness of the sleep lab can therefore be embraced within the poetic enterprise. "There is nothing simultaneously more intimate and more alien," she writes, "than the signal-to-signal readouts of one's own body," a paradox that finds its mirror in the fact that "there is nothing more intimate and more alien than to sleep."[72]

The centrality of the lab thus forms the basis for Huber's experiment with a poetics of sleep, and her approach hinges on the insight, made possible through EEGs and brain science, that sleep is not a single thing. As is well known in the post-EEG world, the process of sleep is not uniform but consists of startlingly different states, "cycled through in ninety-minute intervals from non-REM sleep stages 1 to 2 to 3 and 4 to REM sleep marking the finale before it all starts again."[73] Just as crucially, sleep and waking are not necessarily fully distinct from one another. Studies show that sleep may be local rather than global – that is, "not sweeping throughout the whole organism, the whole brain at once, but occurring in pockets, individual cortical columns or neuronal assemblies."[74] Huber notes that apparently no one with brain damage has ever lost the ability to sleep, which means that sleep does not belong to one particular area of the brain but maintains its presence within whatever neurons survive.[75] Moreover, the transition into sleep tends to be so stealthy that lab patients will often disagree with the machine's report that they were asleep at a given time. In the first stage of sleep, known as non-REM sleep stage 1, if someone "were to ask, 'Are you asleep,' you would answer, 'No.'"[76] The intermingling of sleep and wakefulness thus requires "a complete re-evaluation of what it means to be engaged in either,"[77] and a poetics of sleep must account for this.

A notable feature of Huber's approach is that she rejects traditional poetic representations of sleep in figurative terms. She observes, with some annoyance, that from Greek mythology, through to Shakespeare, up to contemporary poetry, sleep has been associated metaphorically with death. For Huber, this is a tired arrangement that does not reflect the richness and "constant movement" of sleep, especially now that sleep has changed with the knowledge emerging from sleep labs and EEGs.[78] Likewise, literary representations of sleep have often taken dreams as their focus, which, ironically, largely sidesteps a focus on the world of sleep by emphasizing conscious experience and figurative thought. Although Hamlet wonders "in that sleep of death what dreams may come,"[79] such lyricism rarely speaks about sleep *as* sleep, preferring instead to find in sleep a vehicle for figurative visions of death and desire. "At once found everywhere and nowhere in the body," Huber writes, sleep is "everywhere and missing from poetry."[80] She therefore proposes a method of sleep poetics that refuses to engage in sleep as a symbol. "The first thing a poetics can leave behind in movement," Huber concludes, "is the metaphor linking sleep and death. The second thing it can leave behind in movement is metaphor, or any particular literary device altogether."[81]

What remains within a poetics of sleep when we have rejected symbolism must be a kind of contradiction: a literal representation of sleep, accomplished through the inherently symbolic structures of language. For Huber, the EEG provides the model for this impossible task. The EEG "presents itself in the place of metaphor – it says (fallibly, utopically, like any system of writing says), 'I'm not here to make an arbitrary connection, I'm here to show you the thing itself' ... The unbroken trace of electroencephalography is the narrative through which sleep is made recognizable, visible, a machinic cipher of an organic chronicle."[82] Huber, then, is very aware of the impossibility of her project. She will create a poetics of sleep based on the printed graph of an EEG, which itself presumes, absurdly, to represent the reality of sleep on a page.

The second half of *Assembling the Morrow* is Huber's poetry of sleep, which, naturally, is incoherent. Using a copy of her own EEG graph as a template, or "writable vector,"[83] Huber creates nonrepresentational or semi-representational poetry that charts the contours of the EEG, following its peaks and valleys across the page. Excerpts of this poem-chart are presented as a series of foldout pages that extend for three feet when fully opened.

For a nonspecialist reader, the peaks and valleys of the EEG chart are immediately recognizable in the signature shape of the machine brain scan, a notion that is familiar from countless pop culture representations. In an episode of the television series *The Big Bang Theory*, Sheldon (Jim Parsons)

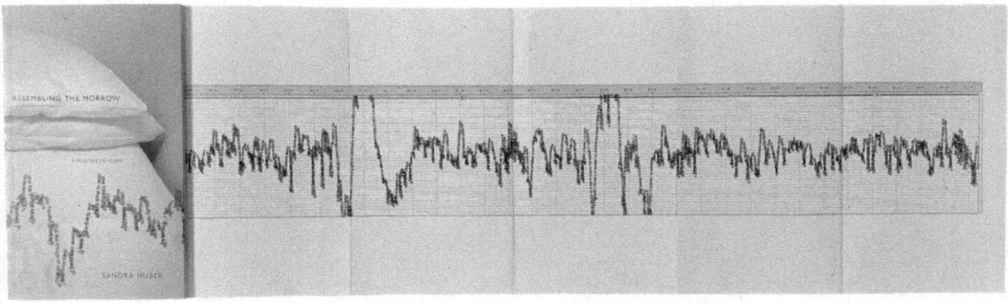

4.2 Sandra Huber, "Non-REM 2 Sleep," 2014.

believes that he can overcome a mental block in his dark matter research by increasing his stress levels, so Amy (Mayim Bialik) connects him to an EEG and experiments with ways to irritate him.[84] In the original *Ghostbusters*,[85] Louis Tully (Rick Moranis) is hooked up to an absurd helmet reminiscent of an EEG electrode cap, which reveals that he has been possessed by Vinz Clortho, the Keymaster of Gozer. Most of us have no idea how to draw any specific meaning from the lines on an EEG, but we understand that the chart is purported to represent, in some objective sense, the "real" operation of the brain – a grandiose claim that makes the machine a good target for satire as well as admiration. The EEG chart is a symbol of arcane knowledge and the dominance of science in revealing the secrets of the human mind.

The EEG poem charts in *Assembling the Morrow* draw on the cultural familiarity of the EEG, preserving the symbolic aspects of the chart as a paradoxical representation of both knowledge and mystery. True to the form of the EEG chart, in which the information presented is both impressively detailed and hopelessly obscure, the written content of Huber's poem is densely arranged but nearly impossible to decipher. Many of the words are not words at all but fragments of words, and even these fragments are usually obscured by further layers of fragments printed one on top of another, as though a child has been playing with a jammed typewriter. In those rare moments when the writing becomes legible – when the line climbs a sudden lengthy peak in the graph, for instance – comprehension seems tantalizingly close but remains stubbornly out of reach. One of the most comprehensible lines in "Non-REM 3 and 4 Sleep" reads: "there e a are e n no o w windows s i in n t this s r room m o of f w walls s." The struggle that we must undergo to

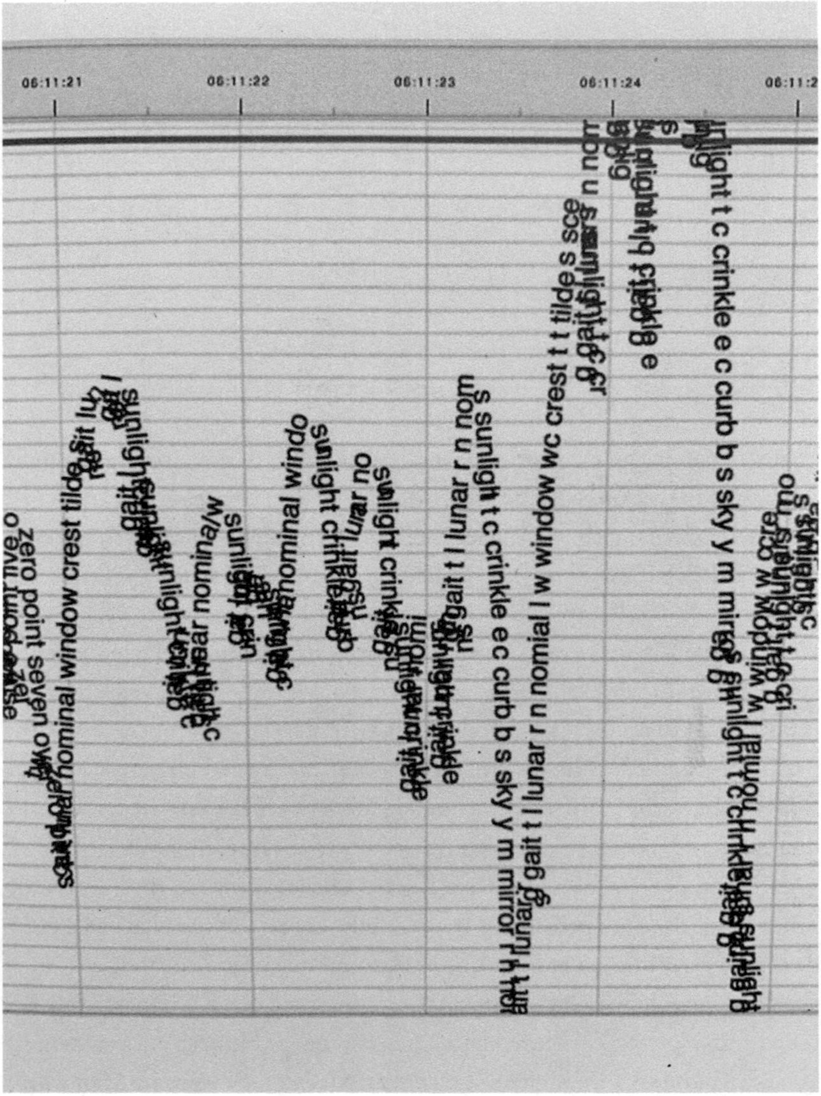

4.3 Text detail of Sandra Huber, "Non-REM 2 Sleep," 2014.

read these lines hints at a deeper struggle within the brain. Huber's sleeping mind wants to establish a sense of meaning through language, but as she remains unable to string words together, the effort to create meaningful syntax is painstaking and tragic.

The book also provides a transcription of the EEG poetry written as a more standard column of text. The transcription runs for some fifty-three pages, although this total represents merely a small excerpt of Huber's project. "There are approximately twenty-four minutes written," she explains, "(or, 241,604 characters, some 300 pages, from 6:11:01 to 6:35:43 a.m.), of which only just over two minutes are presented here."[86] One of the most startling features of this poetry is thus the sheer volume of it. A fifty-three-page transcript that corresponds to two minutes of sleep provides a window into the surprising amount of brain activity that must occur during the course of a night. Even with such a small fraction of the transcript published in the book, only the most patient reader would work their way through line after line of fractured words and broken syntax. A somewhat randomly selected passage reads,

wishingly i
timely t
w
timely
wishingl
tim
wishin
timely t
wishing
time
wishingly i
timely to wonder. i
wishingly i knew
timel
wish
i have time to wo
she has thi
i have time to wonder. i ha
she has things of whi
i
s
i ha[87]

Whereas a true EEG must be deciphered by clinical specialists, Huber's charts, as a product of subjective experience reflected through language, bring the duty of interpretation into the realm of the humanities, yet this relocation of meaning results in texts that can be deciphered by no one. Because the fragments contain tantalizing bits of recognizable speech, they torment and tease the reader with the expectation that, just maybe, something sensible will emerge. The poetry is exasperating because it *almost* means something.

Herein lies one of the contradictions of Huber's project. The charts of poetry are meant to present a vision of sleep that emerges from the sleepside, yet despite (or because of) all the electronic equipment, the impressive technologies of the sleep lab, the vectors, the software, and the hours at the keyboard, what finally emerges is a form of representation that remains stubbornly tied to the waking world. The EEG is a technological apparatus created by and for the waking mind, and the fragments of words in the EEG poetry are broken bits of waking language. Is the experience of sleep really a shattered version of waking life, where "there are no windows" becomes "there e a are e n no o w windows s"? The collapse of meaningful language does indeed suggestively echo the befoggedness of the threshold of sleep, but the difficulty with this act of translation is that it presents sleep not as its own form but as a broken, distorted version of wakefulness. Being only partly facetious, we might say that the project undertaken in *Assembling the Morrow* is reminiscent of the task performed by Satan in *Paradise Lost*, who spends his time perverting and corrupting the goodness of God's creation. Because evil has no true form in and of itself, it can be expressed only through the breaking down of what is divine. Like the fallen angel, Huber's EEG poetry must break apart the goodness of language, filling the page with a corrupted form drawn from waking life, because no sleepside form of representation exists. This approach results in the impression that sleep is a struggle, a hopelessly faulty attempt to mimic waking life. Real sleep, however, isn't a struggle. It's the easiest thing in the world.

Huber is sharply aware of these contradictions. As she observes in an interview, "combining words, which are always awake, with traces of sleep, was my way of entering this space that is neither one or the other."[88] And just as Huber signals her self-consciousness with regard to the impossibility of her project, there is certainly a degree of mischief in the way that she sets up the earnest, scholarly nature of her pursuit with a thoughtful, well-researched essay and then, in sheer audacity, publishes dozens of pages of gibberish. The book falls asleep halfway through, but this sleep is a construct, the experimental literary product of a poet whose eyes are very much open. *Assembling the Morrow* is an ingenious work, and it pushes the asymptotic line closer than ever to the sleepside, but the sleepside remains maddeningly out of reach. If anything, the book heightens the sense in which sleep is unfathomable. The work is as much a comment on the limits of technology, language, and wakefulness as it is on the experience of sleep.

A final question that we might pose of *Assembling the Morrow* has to do with Huber's assertion that a poetics of sleep must emerge from a sleep lab. After all, such an assertion means that the poetry will always be encumbered by the assumptions and limitations of science, forever seeing sleep through EEG-coloured glasses. Not only does this turn toward science mean that the poetry becomes constrained by the peaks and valleys of the chart, but it also makes the prospect of abandoning metaphor more difficult. The EEG has indeed changed the way that sleep is understood, but even scientific visions of sleep, whether expressed through charts, graphs, or writing, inevitably involve translation, representation, and figurative thinking. Seeing the EEG as the primary source of sleep knowledge, the spring from which poetic visions of sleep must emerge, reinforces the configurations of power that Huber's poetry otherwise challenges.

Huber recounts an anecdote about an EEG scientist who, upon entering the sleep lab and seeing the live readout from a patient's brain, comments knowingly on the signature shape of the REM sleep waves on the chart, only to then look up at the actual patient who is wide awake and reading a book.[89] This amusing incident might suggest, perhaps fancifully, that reading, through which we take part in the dream life of literature, is the closest we can come to experiencing sleep while awake. More literally, the striking similarity between REM activity and waking activity in the brain raises a curious point about *Assembling the Morrow*. If a person were to record an EEG of their brain activity during their waking hours, the resulting chart, much like Huber's poetry, would show an astonishing amount of activity that would nevertheless fail to correspond to the actual sensations, thoughts, and experiences that make up the person's consciousness and identity. What would happen if Huber's method were used to create a poetics of the waking mind, exploring the patterns of brain activity that lie beyond what can normally be perceived when our eyes are open? The resulting poem charts might look more or less the same (perhaps with better syntax now and then), leaving the poetics of sleep indistinguishable from a poetics of the daytime EEG.

What is gained from Huber's approach, we might say, is not so much an accurate poetic representation of sleep but more importantly a painfully earned awareness of the epistemological gap between sleep and consciousness. Sleep cannot be congruous with consciousness, and therefore it cannot be congruous with language. Language is our best tool for developing our understanding of things – especially things that resist quantification – yet sleep remains that which we cannot understand because the notion of the self, and its carrying case full of words, cannot enter the realm beyond consciousness. Every step that language tries to take toward the sleepside leaves the sleepside one step away. *Assembling the Morrow* is what happens when the unstoppable force of language meets the immovable object of sleep.

5

Sleeping in the Anthropocene

IN JUNE 2013, unusually heavy rains fell on the foothills of the Rocky Mountains in Alberta and on the prairie communities to the east.[1] Over a span of forty-eight hours, some places received the amount of rain that they would usually get in the entire month of June and then saw double that amount again. Rainfall near the tops of the mountains caused rapid snow melt. Meanwhile, much of the deep soil was still frozen and couldn't absorb water, and the shallower ground was already saturated from earlier spring rains. With nowhere else to go, the raging waters quickly overran the rivers that come down from the mountains toward Canmore, High River, Calgary, and other communities. The Bow River that runs through downtown Calgary peaked at eight times its regular flow rate, flooding neighbourhoods, streets, buildings, critical infrastructure, and parks. "Gather your valuables and go," said Calgary mayor Naheed Nenshi to the people in the evacuation zones.[2]

From our little two-bedroom apartment in Calgary's Beltline neighbourhood, Niki and I scrolled through newsfeeds as reports of the rising flood waters became more dire by the hour. As the evacuation orders spread through downtown and other neighbourhoods that line the river, we sympathized with all those poor people rushing to escape with little notice, on the verge of losing their homes and businesses and everything inside. Looking down from our third-floor balcony at the quiet street that runs past our apartment, we talked about how lucky we were that we didn't live downtown, that the Beltline is separated from the city centre by a series of sloped underpasses that would collect any water runoff, and that we weren't near the smaller

Elbow River that connects with the Bow near the Stampede grounds a couple of kilometres to the east. As anxious new parents with an eight-month-old baby, we couldn't imagine how awful it must be for the families close to the rising water. On the city social media channels, the mandatory evacuation zone spread wider and wider as darkness fell on the city, but we were the lucky ones, calmly turning off the lights and peacefully falling asleep in our own beds.

Around midnight, Niki squeezed my shoulder, waking me up. "We have to go," she said. "We're being evacuated."

What? This didn't make sense. We didn't live close to the rivers. We weren't anywhere near the water. I tried to focus my blurry eyes. How could we evacuate? We don't even have a car! Niki was already packing a go-bag. "We have to call Julie," she said.

Our friends Julie and Chris, living another kilometre farther away from the river than us, suddenly became our only frantic hope. I've always been anxious about asking people for favours, and the thought of waking someone up with a midnight phone call seemed as horrifying to me at that moment as the flood itself. *Maybe I'll take my chances with the water,* I thought. But the evacuation was not optional; we needed help. I dialled the phone. Thankfully, a sleepy Julie picked up.

"My good, good friend, Julie," I said, trying to make light. "Did I ever tell you what a good friend you are?" Not missing a beat, they invited us over to stay. We quickly finished packing, put out extra food and water for our cat – surely, she wouldn't be flooded on the third floor, right? – and headed out to the curb where Julie and Chris arrived shortly to pick us up. Back at their place, they immediately insisted on sleeping, somehow, on their living room couch so that Niki, baby Jamie, and I could take the bedroom. We stayed in their apartment for several days, anxiously watching the news reports and occasionally trekking delicately through the neighbourhood to check on our cat, named Cat. Luckily, our street remained dry, but as the days without power stretched on, our dark apartment became surprisingly alien and cold. Everything in the fridge had to be thrown away.

This was how our family became, for a brief period, climate evacuees in our own city. The lived experience of climate disaster took the form of our own lost sleep: Niki stayed awake for hours checking the evacuation zones, we abandoned our home in the middle of the night, and we in turn disrupted the sleep of our friends, who unexpectedly became our twenty-four-hour disaster response team. Amidst all the flooded homes, the lost lives, the ruined infrastructure, and the $5 billion financial impact of the flood, a few nights of fragile sleep may seem insignificant, yet within this experience of sleeplessness was a glimpse into a world of ever-worsening climate disasters. Niki and I have marvelled at how quickly we went from "Thank goodness this won't affect us" to "We're being evacuated!" For us, this climate-induced disruption of our sleep was a shocking event, the likes of which we had never seen before. Jamie, in contrast, was born into a world where the next climate disaster might always be waiting just outside the door, ready to knock in the middle of the night.

In the first large-scale study "to examine the implications of climate change for human sleep," a team of American researchers in 2017 compared personal sleep surveys from 765,000 people with the corresponding weather records for their cities.[3] Higher body temperatures tend to make sleep more difficult, and sure enough, the study showed that people had more trouble sleeping on the hotter nights. This finding does not bode well for the future, especially since nighttime temperatures are rising more quickly than daytime temperatures. In the United States alone, the researchers calculated, a conservative average increase of 1 degree Celsius would result in "nearly 9 million additional nights of insufficient sleep per month." What is more, as with so many of the impacts of global heating, these kinds of effects are not felt equitably across the population but are several times worse for seniors and people with low incomes.

Although this kind of study can be useful for thinking about average temperatures, my family's brief experience with sleepless nights during the Calgary flood of 2013, which involved imposing on Julie and Chris in the middle of the night, is just one small example of how the disruptions the climate crisis poses to good sleep are not limited to the obvious measure of increasing heat. Climate collapse is characterized not just by rising average temperatures but also by tipping points, cascading effects, and sudden disasters. Fires, floods, dangerous storms, water shortages, poisonous ground-level ozone, and continent-wide clouds of smoke are all arriving faster and with greater severity. Whereas global heating can be measured in terms of increasing average temperatures, the weather in any given location tends to be much more erratic, with some places, such as the Arctic and the Global South, faring worse than others. Events such as the flooding of a third of Pakistan in 2022, which displaced 33 million people, and the years-long drought in the Horn of Africa, which has left over 4 million people in severe humanitarian crisis,[4] go far beyond disrupted sleep, yet sleeplessness is surely one terrible part of them. If an average increase of 1 degree Celsius in the United States is a troubling scenario, what will it mean to see more severe heat waves in Lagos, worsening drought in Yemen, or stronger hurricanes in Haiti?[5] With Canada warming twice as fast as the global average, where will we see the next fires like the ones that ravaged Fort McMurray in 2016 and great swaths of the country in 2023 or the next "hundred-year flood" like the ones that struck Quebec in 2017 and 2019?[6] How can we address the fact that urban heat deaths are strongly correlated to poverty and race?[7] Or that 80 per cent of the people displaced by climate change are women?[8] Calculations of global averages can unintentionally conceal the inequitable chaos of global heating.

There is a sense in which statements about the exceptional nature of climate disasters – "this is the worst flood in fifty years" or "this heat wave has broken a hundred-year record" – can paradoxically reveal a sense of unintentional climate denialism. After all, these statements still see the past as a model for what the present is supposed to look like. In a time of accelerating global heating, however, the weather of years gone by is no longer a reasonable baseline. The forest fire smoke drifting into your bedroom window is not the climax of the story of wildfires; it is one step on the path toward ever-more-dizzying climate cruelty. A sad truth of our time is that every climate disaster, no matter how terrible, is a preview of worse ones to come. Let us stop pretending that intense heat waves are the "new normal." Even the most blistering, deadly heat event is always merely a precursor. Even if we stopped burning fossil fuels today, we are locked into a years-long delay between carbon emissions and the resulting heat. The best we can say is that this escalation doesn't have to go on forever; we can begin to slow it down.

Several years after the flooding in Calgary, my family had a glimpse into the terrifying intensity of a supercharged heat wave. In June 2021, a severe heat dome lumbered onto Canada's west coast, bringing previously unimaginable temperatures to British Columbia, Alberta, and the northwestern United States. As is becoming common with climate change, the weather system became stuck in place, pumping hotter and hotter temperatures down onto the Okanagan, Edmonton, Portland, and hundreds of other communities, including Vancouver, where we were located at the time. Whereas the heat waves of the twentieth century would have afforded some relief with lower temperatures at night, the heat dome was relentless, keeping temperatures dangerously high both night and day, one day after another.

Taking shelter from the extreme heat, we cranked up the portable air conditioner in our living room, made plenty of ice cubes, and waited for the heat dome to break. The cool air from the air conditioner was escaping down the hallway, so we pinned heavier and heavier blankets up over the gaps. This jury-rigged system kept the living room only about 4 degrees Celsius cooler than the sweltering kitchen and bedrooms, but those 4 degrees felt like the difference between surviving on our own or having to call the paramedics. A "normal" hot day in Vancouver might reach around 30 degrees, but we watched in horror as the humidex reading rose into the high 30s, the low 40s, and then the high 40s, with warnings of an impending 50 degrees. This was deadly weather. We dragged our mattresses into the living room, our small bubble of survivability, and spent several days doing little else than sitting and drinking water, sleeping fitfully on our improvised beds, and occasionally venturing into the sauna-like kitchen to collect food. In the evening, Jamie would brush half his teeth in the searingly hot bathroom, come back to the living room to recover, and then journey into the bathroom again to finish brushing. This continued for four days and four nights, and we explained to our four-year-old daughter, Holly, that sometimes the weather gets very hot, so we just have to wait. Like Jamie, she will always have lived in a world of climate emergency.

As with the 2013 flood, we were again ultimately among the lucky ones, as our struggling air conditioner created a relatively safe little zone in our otherwise roasting household. Many people were not so fortunate. The village of Lytton broke Canada's all-time high temperature record (previously 45 degrees) with a scorching temperature of 46.6, followed over the next two days by new records of 47.9 and 49.6.[9] The day after that, Lytton burned almost entirely to the ground.[10] Earlier the same month, the Canadian Institute for Climate Choices, a federally funded independent research partnership, had released a report called *The Health Costs of Climate Change: How Canada Can Adapt, Prepare, and Save Lives*. The report cautioned that, by 2050, extreme heat in Canada could cause roughly 300 to 400 deaths per year.[11] When the heat dome struck just one week after the release of the report, the extreme heat killed 619 people in British Columbia alone over a period of seven days, making it the deadliest weather event in Canadian history.[12] And the disasters keep accelerating; a few months after the heat dome, swaths of British Columbia were submerged in catastrophic "once in a century" flooding.[13] Two years later, the province saw its most destructive wildfire season on record so far.[14]

In such situations, saving lives and homes is the urgent priority, yet the problem of sleep will increasingly become a nightly struggle for billions of people throughout this century and beyond. The report from the Canadian Institute for Climate Choices did not mention sleep as a health concern associated with climate change, but sleep is a genuine problem for those who are stuck inside a heat wave or seeking shelter during an evacuation. As the heat dome event unfolded on the ground, news articles remarked that the heat was not only causing heatstroke and dehydration; it was also causing significant problems with people's sleep. Dr Wendy Hall, a sleep expert at the University of British Columbia, explained that "our core body temperature needs to cool down as we get closer to sleeping, but due to this heat wave, our temperatures are staying elevated which makes it much harder to fall asleep."[15] The quality of sleep is affected, too, as an overly warm sleeper will get less deep sleep and less REM time.[16] This is not even to speak of the insomnia that many people endure due to climate anxiety or of the sleeplessness associated with climate-related post-traumatic stress disorder, such as that experienced by survivors of the 2016 fire in Fort McMurray.[17] By imposing more and more severe sleep disruptions, a hotter planet creates a population with reduced learning abilities, poor emotional regulation, and damaged immune systems, harming exactly those capacities that are crucial for adaptation and collective survival. It has become a dark truism, each sweltering summer, for people to remark, "This is the coldest summer for the next 10,000 years." As my family lay awake on those June nights, trapped inside the awful heat dome, I couldn't help wondering: is this the best sleep for the next 10,000 years?

The death toll and massive health costs of intense heat should tell us that air conditioning now needs to be seen as a basic utility, like plumbing and heat. That indoor cooling remains too expensive for many people is just one measure of climate injustice. Even so, no amount of air conditioning can allow people to sleep at ease through a fire, a flood, or a food and water shortage. In 1987, in protest against the colonization of Indigenous land, the Australian band Midnight Oil sang, "How do we sleep while our beds are burning?"[18]

In 2013, their song was rerecorded by an ensemble of celebrities, this time as a protest against carbon emissions and climate change,[19] reminding us that the stability needed for peaceful sleep and peaceful lives is being eroded in an ever widening circle, starting with Indigenous land and now expanding even to the air-conditioned homes that reside on that land.

Although mindfulness phone apps and luxury mattresses might promise to give us a better sleep through consumer spending, taking strong action against global heating is one of the best ways to help us sleep easier over the long term, both figuratively and literally. What is more, as Julie and Chris showed us, fighting the climate crisis isn't just a matter of cutting fossil fuel use or building bigger levees, as crucial as those things are. It's also a matter of caring deeply for others, even to the point, sometimes, of sharing our beds. In their own recollection of the Calgary flood, Julie says that it could just as easily have been them landing on our doorstep that night. They tell us that, far from imposing on them, we gave them the chance to feel hopeful about how we can all collectively take care of one another in an uncertain future.

TALES OF SLEEPLESS WONDER

One of the key lessons of the fight against global heating is that scientific reports are not enough to bring about change. The scientific case for cutting greenhouse gas emissions was established many decades ago, but the collective force of imagination necessary to comprehend climate chaos and to make big social changes has been slow to catch up. We can and should collect mountains of data about the problem, but learning to absorb and address a crisis is a matter of culture, not just information. If we want to learn how to approach sleep in the age of climate collapse, one option would be to wait until just about everyone has learned to endure, first-hand, the sleeplessness brought about by fire evacuations, heat domes, and floods. A much better option is to see how various forms of imaginative representation can reshape our thinking.

Much like actual sleep in the midst of global heating, the representation of sleep in climate fiction has received scant critical attention. Probably the best-known sleeper in Canadian speculative fiction is Snowman in Margaret Atwood's novel *Oryx and Crake*. Snowman is one of the last survivors after human society collapses due to a genetically engineered pandemic virus. The first line of the novel – "Snowman wakes before dawn"[20] – has Snowman resting awkwardly in a tree somewhere near the former Canada-US border, failing to sleep very well as the sun begins to peek up from between the half-submerged crumbling skyscrapers. The horizon is "lit now with a rosy, deadly glow. Strange how that colour still seems tender."[21] The sun is a lethal figure throughout the novel, one of the deadly hazards that Snowman must avoid, along with the vicious wild animals that roam the land. "The sea is hot metal," the narrator observes, "the sky a bleached blue, except for the hole burnt in it by the sun."[22] And later, when "[t]he sun is well up," we are told that "[h]e'd better hurry, or he'll fry."[23] Even the postapocalyptic name that he has given himself, Snowman, refers to a figure that has been driven to extinction by heat. The story's emphasis on genetically engineered posthumans and bizarre hybrid animals makes it read like extravagant science fiction, but Snowman's deadly fear of the sun at such a northern latitude and his inability to sleep well due to its blazing intensity at dawn certainly read like realist fiction now, even if they seemed dystopian back in 2003.

Interestingly, the opening scene of *Oryx and Crake*, where the unbearable rise of the sun prevents Snowman from sleeping, is echoed in the opening scene of American author Kim Stanley Robinson's realist climate novel *The Ministry for the Future*. Here, the protagonist, Frank May, finds himself in a terrible heat wave in a town in the state of Uttar Pradesh in northern India. Early in the morning, Frank looks around at the "square apartment blocks like the one he was in, rooftop patios occupied by residents who had moved up there in the night, it being too hot to sleep inside. Now quite a few of them were standing behind their chest-high walls looking east ... Frank took a deep breath. It reminded him of the air in a sauna. This the coolest part of the day ... And then the sun cracked the eastern horizon. It blazed like an atomic bomb, which of course it was."[24] Wailing cries soon fill the air, as "people were discovering sleepers in distress, finding those who would never wake up from the long hot night."[25] As the sun rises higher and hotter in the sky, Robinson develops one of the most horrific and unforgettable scenes in modern fiction; the heat and humidity produce a "wet-bulb" temperature at which the human body can no longer cool itself through the evaporation of water from the skin. Without the ability to regulate their body temperatures through sweating, people simply stop moving and die. Those who are still alive crawl desperately into the lake, which seems like the right thing to do, except that the water has risen above body temperature. Sitting helpless in the lake with all the others, with nowhere to escape to, Frank "had a thirst that couldn't be slaked. Hot water in one's stomach meant there was no refuge anywhere, the world both inside and outside well higher than human body temperature ought to be. They were being poached."[26] As day turns to night, the old people die, the young people die, and then the strong and healthy people die. "Many years passed for Frank that night," and finally he is all alone in the midst of death.[27] Of these two climate fictions, both of which open with scenes of broken sleep during hot nights, *Oryx and Crake* is the outlandish sci-fi story, yet it is Robinson's realist scene that is more shocking, more horrendous, more repulsive to the imagination.

Despite their very different approaches to imagining global heating, both *Oryx and Crake* and *The Ministry for the Future*, like many works of climate fiction, portray the lived experience of the climate crisis as something that belongs primarily to the future, whether that future is imagined through a dystopian fantasy or through a more realist speculation. This focus creates a potential problem, as the very notion of climate fiction as a genre seems to assume that climate change is a speculative scenario, and thus, ironically, there is a sense in which cli-fi novels risk downplaying the fact that climate change has been a present-day experience for quite some time, particularly for marginalized people in vulnerable regions.

In his influential book *The Great Derangement: Climate Change and the Unthinkable*, Amitav Ghosh develops an extended complaint about the apparent inability of narrative fiction to portray the era of climate chaos. He argues that because the English tradition of literary novels has always been centred on the notion of the individual protagonist, the novel form is poorly suited to represent the large-scale problems of the Anthropocene. This failure of the dominant literary imagination, Ghosh says, "will have to be counted as an aspect of the broader imaginative and cultural failure that lies at the heart of the climate crisis."[28] One of the obvious rebuttals to Ghosh's position is that speculative fiction is exactly the genre that *can* represent the age of ecological collapse. Ghosh, however, anticipates this argument and dismisses speculative genres very quickly:

> Is it the case that science fiction is better equipped to address the Anthropocene than mainstream literary fiction? This might appear obvious to many. After all, there is now a new genre of science fiction called "climate fiction" or cli-fi. But cli-fi is made up mostly of disaster stories set in the future, and that, to me, is exactly the rub. The future is but one aspect of the Anthropocene: this era also includes the recent past, and, most significantly, the present ... [The Anthropocene] is precisely not an imagined "other" world apart from ours; nor is it located in another "time" or another "dimension." By no means are the events of the era of global warming akin to the stuff of wonder tales.[29]

Ghosh's rejection of works that take place in the future because they don't take place in the present seems ungenerous, a bit like criticizing Dickens's *Oliver Twist* for focusing on exploitative child labour in England rather than looking at labour troubles overseas. Most of the effects of climate change *do* belong to the future, even if present-day experiences and the floods and fires in the rearview mirror are already truly awful. Moreover, with climate change, the present and the future tend to blur together as disasters accelerate, so writing about the future is a sensible way of coming to terms with the present. If Ghosh wants to read novels that deal with global heating in our own present-day reality, such as Barbara Kingsolver's *Flight Behavior*, he is free to do so, or indeed to write such novels himself, which he has done. There is room at the table for many kinds of stories. For my purposes, Atwood and Robinson both succeed, in a very visceral way, in helping our imaginations to recognize how global heating affects sleep, a factor that scientific and policy approaches have often neglected.

Moreover, the value of speculative writing is not limited to novels but also emerges through other forms such as short stories. We might consider, for instance, Christiane Vadnais's short story collection *Fauna* (*Faunes* in the original French), which won the City of Quebec book award and the Horizons Imaginaires speculative fiction award in 2019. *Fauna* is a series of linked stories about a world ravaged by global heating and catastrophic floods, and sure enough, sleep in this book is not restful. Before the stories even get underway, the collection opens with a glimpse of troubled slumbers: "Just like their prehistoric ancestors, human beings still dream at night of epic fights with animals ... Outstretched arms serve not to embrace the sleeping body at their side but to fend off wolves and bears."[30] In one of the stories in the volume, people in a makeshift village sleep in tents fashioned from old ships' sails.[31] The evocative image of the sails, which are meant to travel on the wind but now sit stationary, implies that the dreams and slumbers that take place within them must also have been repurposed to enable survival in a harsh new reality. In another story, civilization crumbles due to an epidemic caused by a parasitic crustacean unleashed by climate change, and a group of infected people wait restlessly to die, "punching themselves in the stomach at night ... in the hope of injuring the interloper within."[32] The deranged self-harm that makes sleep impossible calls to mind the desperate sense of helplessness that might often be said to characterize life under climate change. "Like every other facet of their lives," Vadnais writes, "their insomnia is collective."[33] *Fauna* was published in 2018, just prior to the arrival of Covid-19, and the collection's nightmarish linking of ecological trouble with pandemics now seems horribly prescient. That the stories take place in a time that is not quite our own should hardly be held against them. In her commentary on speculative writing, Diletta De Cristofaro notes that novels that imagine a future without sleep tend to overlap with climate fiction in telling ways. "A powerful environmental thread," she writes, "also runs through many of these fictions, in which climate-breakdown Earth is paralleled with human bodies breaking down under the weight of constant hyper-vigilance."[34] Although her observation may apply most obviously to novels such as *The Marrow Thieves* (discussed in chapter 3), it can also illuminate works of other kinds, such as *Fauna*. Stories about a world without sleep may take place in another dimension, but like all good fictions, they have much to say about the anxieties and hopes of our own world.

Nevertheless, Ghosh's critique is hard to put out of one's mind when reading works of cli-fi, especially in terms of the politics of environmental racism. The climate disasters of the first decades of the twenty-first century have often been felt most deeply by Indigenous Peoples, citizens of the Global South, and those who are marginalized due to poverty and race. Looking at the issue in a longer historical context, environmental humanities scholar Pamela Banting argues that "there are two non-concurrent Anthropocenes in Canada. Indigenous people in Canada have been living in one that can be clocked back to more than four hundred years ago, while a second one is looming that has only just begun to afflict non-indigenous Canadians."[35] This second wave of the Anthropocene is of course the one that is recognized in dominant discourse. There is an uncomfortable sense in which speculative narratives such as *Oryx and Crake, The Ministry for the Future,* and others such as Nathaniel Rich's *Odds against Tomorrow,* all written by successful white authors, are consistent with the idea that climate and environmental disasters become remarkable or real only when they happen to financially comfortable white people. In *The Ministry for the Future,* the scene where the American character Frank emerges from the lake as the lone survivor after all the Uttar Pradesh locals have died is certainly unsettling in its racial tropes. The narrative function of the Indian townspeople is to die off in the first chapter in order to establish the terrors of high wet-bulb temperatures – we see their "brown faces flushed red with heat" as they cook in the lake[36] – whereas Frank's survival is required because it is his story that Robinson wants to tell.

Later in his novel, Robinson develops a much broader interest in diverse characters, regions, and inequities, with the result that pinning down a final analysis of the story's tropes becomes pleasingly difficult. Ultimately, it isn't so much that these kinds of stories are doing something wrong but that we need to read beyond them. The risks involved in reading a narrow set of speculative novels is similar, in a way, to the risk of my relating my personal account of the Alberta floods; the story can work if it opens up into larger concerns, but seems foolish if it's just about me. A fuller sense of the complexity and nuance afforded by speculative fiction comes about when reading works – *The Marrow Thieves,* for instance – by a greater diversity of authors. Larissa Lai's genre-bending novel *Salt Fish Girl,* set in 2044 in a watery area previously known as Vancouver, takes a surreal but illuminating interest in the past, present, and future. The protagonist Miranda suffers from a "dreaming disease," whose victims must endure the awful cruelty of remembering events from before they were born. One girl with the disease "remembered all the wars ever fought. She could recall and recount every death, every rape, every wound, every moment of suffering that had ever been inflicted by a member of her ancestral lineage."[37] Miranda finds that the disease makes her talk in her sleep. "It was terribly upsetting," she says, "to think that my parents might know what I dreamt at night."[38] In a story about goddesses and genetically engineered part-humans, the notion of distressed sleep as a prominent theme is perhaps unexpected, but then again, why should we not expect troubles with sleep to characterize a world of gated communities, technological inequity, legacies of trauma, and rising seas? Although Ghosh's comments are useful for thinking about how to read beyond speculative or fantastical works, the novels that he dismisses as "wonder tales" have rich potential for helping us to imaginatively think through the meanings of social fragility and ecological collapse in our present time and beyond.

Pitting Anthropocene novels about the future against those that take place in the present, then, creates a false choice. Moreover, another useful way to respond to Ghosh's critique is to step around it by remembering that novels and short stories are not the only game in town when it comes to narrative arts and figurative representation. What might we say about the thoughtful representation of the present in collections of poetry such as Alice Major's *Welcome to the Anthropocene*? Just as importantly, the desire to find literary works that "address" the Anthropocene seems inherently suspicious. The idea that a great work of literature can represent "the human experience" has been debunked; diverse people face endlessly complex and inequitable conditions, and a refusal to recognize this fact has often gone hand in hand with the creation of long lists of canonical texts by white male writers. Understanding the imaginative force of diverse human experiences is a perpetual process that requires encountering many kinds of works and voices. Surely, the same must be true of representing the Anthropocene, which is, after all, an umbrella term for the entire roiling ocean of events unfolding in our own time and the times to come. Representing the Anthropocene cannot be a matter solely of focusing on big, obvious climate disasters, as important as those events are. We need to consider imaginative reflections of all kinds.

SLEEPING ON A STRANGE PLANET

Sleep appears to be over half a billion years old, having evolved through invertebrate marine creatures before making its way, much later, into larger animals such as mammals and birds.[39] Even bacteria, which evolved further back in time, have circadian cycles that follow the planet's daily sequence of light and darkness.[40] Similar cycles occur in algae, fungi, and plants, and indeed they are seen within individual cells across perhaps all organisms.[41] German forester and ecological writer Peter Wohlleben claims that the winter dormancy of deciduous trees is a form of sleep and that an oak tree planted in a container in your living room will likely die from sleep deprivation.[42] Slumber and similar cyclical patterns exist in a web that binds together most of the species on earth.

Despite its deep evolutionary origins, however, sleep is by no means uniform. Different species sleep for very different amounts of time and in different ways. Elephants sleep for around two hours a night, whereas little brown bats sleep for nineteen hours.[43] When mallard ducks sleep in a row, the outermost birds keep half of their brains awake so they can watch for predators to either side.[44] Dolphins, too, "can sleep with one half of their brain at a time, while the other half stays alert."[45] Researchers have found that octopuses, like humans, alternate between active and quiet stages of sleep, which suggests that they may have gained REM-like sleep, and perhaps even the ability to dream, through an evolutionary line independent from our own.[46] Moreover, as sociologist Eric L. Hsu argues, the sleep of nonhuman animals "is also a sociological matter."[47] He points to how humans make culturally significant choices about co-sleeping with some animals but not others, how the nighttime habits of cats and dogs can keep exhausted pet owners awake at night, and how the daytime drowsiness of nocturnal animals can frustrate customers at zoos who want to be entertained during the day.[48] Despite intensive human control over other species, animals can still sleep in "socially unsettling ways."[49]

Human sleep is tied to the ecological world not just through the rising and setting of the sun or through companionship with restless cats and dogs but also through endless forms of interrelatedness. Circadian rhythms must adapt to location and season since the day-night cycle looks very different at the equator, for instance, than it does in an Arctic summer. The ecosystem finds its way into our bedrooms through the use of cotton in bed sheets and feathers in pillows. When sleep-deprived commuters make their way to work in the morning, they rely on carbon-intensive supply chains that bring coffee beans from tropical plantations to Tim Hortons, where the beans are infused into disposable cups. Recent studies have found not only that human sleep undergoes seasonal changes (with more REM sleep in the winter, for example) but also that our sleep habits tend to be synchronized with lunar phases, such that people sleep significantly less during the nights leading up to the full moon; surprisingly, this lunar alignment has held true both for university students in the urban centre of Seattle and for members of rural Indigenous communities in Argentina.[50] Historian Sasha Handley, a leading expert on sleep practices in early modern England, has been working with postdoctoral fellows to examine how sleep practices have been tied to environmental conditions such as climate, diet, the use of botanicals, and the demands of agricultural labour.[51] Fossilized human remains in Spain show evidence that early humans may have actually hibernated to survive harsh winters.[52] Our bodies even form their own ecosystems of sleep, as parasites within our microbiomes can operate on their own intrinsic circadian rhythms that are "independent of the host."[53] One such parasite is *Trypanosoma brucei*, the unicellular protist that causes human sleeping sickness.[54] Sleep is always a tangled collection of experiences across humans and other species.

These are just some of the ways that the ecological dimensions of sleep extend beyond the matter of climate change. Nevertheless, in concert with capitalism and technology, the complexities of global heating remain central for understanding the nuanced and unequal implications of modern sleep. Jonathan Crary argues that the notion of the 24/7 society that never sleeps "is inseparable from environmental catastrophe in its declaration of permanent expenditure, of endless wastefulness for its sustenance, in its terminal disruption of the cycles and seasons on which ecological integrity depends."[55] Benjamin Reiss similarly finds that "the forces damaging sleep over the past two centuries are the same ones despoiling our ecological system to this day."[56] He notes that waking up before sunrise in the winter requires extra energy consumption, that pharmaceutical sleep chemicals flow from our bodies into the water supply, that "we train our children to sleep in separate bedrooms, thereby requiring larger homes with larger carbon footprints," and that the very notion of making sleep conform to modern cultural standards requires "an attitude of dominion over nature (including our own bodies) through technology and consumerism."[57] Even when people take action to move toward better sustainability – by replacing sodium streetlights with more efficient LEDs, for instance – sleep can be affected in unexpected ways. Because LED light tends to be more blue-tinted than the orange glow of sodium lamps, energy-efficient lighting is now causing melatonin suppression, sleep loss, and nighttime behavioural changes in humans, animals, and insects.[58] Such problems should not be taken as meaning that efforts toward sustainability are undertaken in vain but that the ecological complexities of sleep require a great deal of ongoing attention. Sleeping in the Anthropocene is a matter of accounting for the upheavals of the climate crisis and environmental collapse as well as for the long evolutionary lineage of diverse ecological approaches to sleep on a spinning planet.

POETRY AS SLEEP

Literature and art can offer a way to connect these threads, showing how we might conceive of sleep in relation to climate change, social inequities, the modern capitalist economy, and a sense of connection to specific environments. Here, I consider three examples of how such ecological readings of sleep can take shape, emerging from three very different forms: poetry, temporary "landwork" photography, and comics. In their diversity, these works show how the business of thinking through sleep in the Anthropocene cannot be reduced to a singular vision or framework. In their specificity, each text proposes its own model for developing a literacy of sleep in a world of ecological and cultural complexity, hazards, and beauty.

Poet and professor Rita Wong is well known for her decolonial writing and activism, particularly in regard to the protection of water on Indigenous land. Her poem "sleepless in Somba K'e," from her collection *undercurrent*, takes place in the Northwest Territories where the Yellowknife River flows into Yellowknife Bay at Great Slave Lake. The poem is dedicated to the river itself – "*for the Coney River, otherwise known as the Yellowknife River*" – on the home of the Wiliideh Yellowknives Dene First Nation.[59] This place is, she writes,

> precariously perched on once-infinite ice & sweltering in broken records so many degrees of industry intrusion on the front lines of global ~~warming~~ dying
>
> ...
>
> illuminated by the midnight sun, you flow regardless of the Giant Gold Mine's steady leak of 237,000 tonnes of arsenic trioxide, the bustle of unionized Ekati diamond mine workers, the repeated dramas of visitors, hunters, bureaucrats, researchers, tourists, more miners, students
>
> Snap Lake is "Canada's first completely underground diamond mine."
> after the unsettlers are finished, what legacy will it leave?[60]

With the river carrying toxins leached from the gold and diamond mines and with the ice disappearing as the North heats up more rapidly than the rest of the planet, the term "sleepless" in the title of the poem speaks to the anxiety, frustration, and fear brought about due to the ecological destruction wreaked by industry. The Giant Gold Mine operated in Yellowknife from 1948 to 2004, during which time it did indeed produce "237,000 tonnes of arsenic trioxide dust, making it one of the largest stored arsenic sites in the world."[61] This dust has created awful toxic contamination and long-term remediation problems; the arsenic is being stored underground, but its containment depends on the stability of the permafrost, which is now melting, requiring that new experimental containment methods be put in place.[62] Snap Lake, meanwhile, a diamond mine owned by De Beers, was closed five years after the publication of Wong's poem, partly because "the company was unable to address ongoing issues of meeting water quality standards set for the underground mine," again creating a long-term remediation problem.[63] The title of Wong's poem alludes to the romantic comedy film *Sleepless in Seattle*,[64] but the light-hearted courtship of actors Meg Ryan and Tom Hanks is pointedly replaced here by the atrocities of colonization in the form of industrial poisoning and global heating. The poem takes the problem of insomnia, portrayed as a figure of comedy in the Hollywood movie, and shows that for those who face the consequences of the settler society's actions, sleeplessness is a much more literal and serious matter.

The river is also sleepless given that it is "illuminated by the midnight sun" due to its northern latitude. The two forms of sleeplessness in the poem, one associated with the anxiety of environmental destruction and the other with patterns of daylight in subarctic regions, draw a conceptual link between ecological damage and the North. The city of Yellowknife is not quite northern enough to have a true midnight sun, although the sky does remain illuminated when the sun dips briefly below the horizon on the summer solstice. The persistence of sunlight, which makes sleeping very difficult, thus comes to symbolize the insomnia-causing anxiety that hangs figuratively in the air in the form of poisoned rivers and the vanishing of northern ways of life.

A more positive ecological vision of sleep emerges in the next poem in *undercurrent*, titled "what remains," which begins:

sleep replenishes
a tired mind
birdsong renews
wild life in city's midst[65]

Juxtaposition is the most economical way to create a metaphor. Here, the sleep that replenishes a tired mind is placed immediately before the birdsong that renews "wild life" in the city, creating a conceptual link through which we see birdsong as sleep and, perhaps, sleep as birdsong. The technique is the same one made famous in English by Ezra Pound in his poem "In a Station of the Metro":

The apparition of these faces in the crowd:
Petals on a wet, black bough.[66]

With no verb connecting the two fragments, Pound's short poem creates a metaphorical link between the petals and the faces through their juxtaposition, helped along by the colon at the end of the first line, which clarifies that the two images are both separated and connected. Wong abstains from the colon, allowing the simple juxtaposition and the line breaks to do the work. Birdsong, the metaphor says, plays the same replenishing role as sleep, doing so for the ecosystem in the city rather than for the mind. This role, in turn, creates a secondary metaphor of ecosystem as mind. Just as the mind is a complex network of living activity that requires recovery from exhaustion, the wild environment needs to recover from its depletion due to oppressive human activity in the city. This poem thus forms a companion piece to "sleepless in Somba K'e." Whereas one of the poems draws an association between ecological harm and insomnia, the other one links ecological recovery with the replenishment of sleep. The use of birdsong at the heart of this renewal also nods self-consciously to the role that poetry plays in witnessing and responding to ecological relations. Birds and their songs are iconic metaphors for poetry, a creative form through which the imagination takes flight in language. Poetry, too, is a kind of sleep, a fertile realm beyond usual consciousness through which we can relate to our ecological worlds with fresh eyes.

In the previous chapter, I considered Sandra Huber's complaint that poets tend to use sleep as a symbolic figure – an image of death or desire – rather than investigating the experience of sleep itself. Thinking about poetic visions of sleep and the environment might inspire us to approach this problem from a different angle. Poet Don McKay, who has written thoughtfully about the difficulty of representing "nature" in language, has observed that although Romantic poetry is often seen as nature poetry, it tends to represent nature as a figure of human poetic inspiration rather than *as* nature.[67] For McKay, true nature poetry comes about when the poet operates from an unexpected definition of "wilderness." Wilderness, he proposes, is "the capacity of all things to elude the mind's appropriations."[68] When something surprises us in a way that escapes our expectations or sense of ownership, wilderness becomes visible. This deceptively simple definition has wide-ranging implications for how we understand not only the environment but also culture, language, and thought. You might consider how you can identify wilderness in the ragged edge of a fingernail or in a moment when you struggle to find the right words. One effect of McKay's notion of wilderness is that it confounds the usual distinction between nature and culture, allowing us to comprehend wilderness as a quality that exists, to one degree or another, in everything.

What does this vision of wilderness have to do with sleep? Well, it tells us that poetry about sleep *is* nature poetry. Thoughtful poems can try to represent the wilderness of sleep, a realm that sparks astonishment and escapes the appropriations of the mind. This capacity of poetry also means that eradicating figurative thinking from a poetics of sleep doesn't need to be the goal. Rita Wong's poems, for example, are illuminating largely because they understand sleep in both literal and figurative terms. Her poems do engage with sleep *as* sleep, yet they also recognize that because sleep always occurs within a particular context – alongside a warming northern river contaminated with industrial pollution or within a city where pavement becomes ecosystem – sleep necessarily carries meaning, associative links, and figurative weight. As good students of wilderness, we, too, can consider how sleep, that wild ecosystem of the mind, takes shape at the intersection of the literal and the symbolic.

SLEEPING PLACES AND NO-SLEEPING PLACES

Marlene Creates is an environmental artist whose photography and temporary "landworks" have been exhibited across Canada and around the world for nearly fifty years. One of her best-known installations is *Sleeping Places, Newfoundland 1982*, a collection of twenty-five black and white photos, each one showing a different patch of ground where Creates slept as she travelled around Newfoundland for two months. Each photo shows a faint impression of Creates's body – a small hollow of rumpled ferns, tall grasses, or tiny blossoms upon which she spent the night. In some photos the indentations are obvious patches of crushed and swirled stalks surrounded by tall upright grass that remains untouched, while other photos require some squinting and guesswork to figure out where the impression of her body begins and ends among the stubby ground cover. The photos don't reproduce well in small form, but the picture in your mind is already pretty accurate.

An odd thing about the photos, which are tightly cropped and shot looking straight down, is that they provide no context. Is this patch of grass in the middle of a sweeping field? On the edge of a small clearing? Within sight of the ocean? In an overgrown lot? Creates notes that she spent her nights "on the barrens," but this isn't much to go on. And this lack of specificity, certainly, is part of the point. "The land has a memory," Creates writes in her artist's statement. "The night I spent on the barrens, which felt like the middle of nowhere, the spot where I slept became a place to me."[69] This comment brings to mind another of McKay's idiosyncratic definitions, this time of the word "place." Wondering how we might define place not in the usual terms of home or nation but "as a function of wilderness," McKay writes,

> Try this: "place is wilderness to which history has happened." Or: "place is land to which we have occurred." This would involve asking, for example, not "what's the beach to me?" but "what am I to the beach?" Our occurrence to the land – the act which makes place place – could be a major change (homestead, development, resource extraction) or a smaller claim (prospector's stake, survey marker, plastic tape, souvenir stone), but it shifts the relationship; it brings the wild area into the purview of knowledge and makes it – perhaps momentarily, perhaps permanently – a category of mind.[70]

For Creates, a small patch of anonymous grass becomes a place through the act of sleep. Sleeping on a piece of land "wakes" that land up, as it were, and grants it a sense of character as place, removing it from what we had perceived (or not bothered to perceive) as its anonymity. In this sense the title of the installation turns two ways: Creates is sleeping in these places, and the little patches of ground are sleeping – not yet made into places – until Creates arrives.

In the physical impression of her body on the ground, Creates and the land share a vulnerability. She has let her body drift into sleep in a precarious position outdoors, exposed to the wind and weather without even a tent. (Did she at least use a sleeping bag? We can't tell.) The grasses and ferns, meanwhile, have been crushed by her weight in one small area, forcing them to become a place that carries meaning for Creates and for the viewers of her photographs due to the fact that they are damaged. In his comments on the photos, British nature writer Robert Macfarlane notes that "there is something creaturely to them ... yet they are also oddly, quietly disturbing. The heart of every image glows a spectral silver from the extra light reflected by the flattened blades of grass or the pressed-down fern leaves ... At the edges of each mute image presses a sense of exposure, tending to danger."[71] Part of this haunting sense of exposure lies in the fact that the impression of Creates's sleep, the transformation of wilderness into place, is only momentary. The indentation will quickly fade, and once Creates walks away, she will probably never again be able to find the place where she slept. Certainly, no one else could. This fact also lends the images a sense of nostalgia and affection; these places have nurtured Creates's sleep through their placeness, coming into existence only to say farewell as soon as the sleep has ended. By pointing the camera straight down from eye level, Creates directs our focus to a minute patch that holds meaning solely through the interaction between her sleeping body and the grass, not through the usual elements of scenery – the landmarks, grand vistas, and street signs – that normally register as place. The act of sleep and the framing of the photograph around its imprint fill up one small piece of "barren" land.

One can imagine some alternative approaches that Creates could have taken to this project, such as simply walking up to a piece of ground and taking its photo without bothering with the sleep. Missing from such a photograph would be the sense of intimacy, care, and relationship that comes about through physical closeness with the land and through the vulnerability of lying down and allowing consciousness to drift away. Likewise, a more intrusive approach would have resulted in a different kind of work altogether. Creates notes, about her earlier photography project involving long strips of crisp white paper laid along the ground, that she conceived of this work "in deliberate opposition to large-scale earthworks – high-impact interventions made in the land with excavators and bulldozers in the 1960s and '70s – mostly by male artists in the United States. As a young artist (twenty-seven years old), I didn't have the courage to verbalize this and challenge artworks that were celebrated at the time. What I said was, 'With the paper I was able to make a simple gesture which left no permanent mark.' The non-monumental has preoccupied me since then."[72] In *Sleeping Places*, the creation of a mark or gesture makes the place *her* patch of land, but contrary to the industrial-sized earthworks, this sense of connection is notable primarily for being momentary and subtle. When she walks away from her place of sleep, she gives the land back to the wilderness.

McKay engaged explicitly with *Sleeping Places, Newfoundland 1982* in 2012 with the publication of his ekphrastic poem "Sleeping Places," which reflects on the representation of land in Creates's installation. The poem portrays sleep as a form of writing, a gesture that turns the land, only briefly, into a medium for human concerns. Creates's photos, the poem suggests, portray a "plot," both in the sense of a demarcated piece of land and in the sense of a narrative. In each of these senses, the photos emphasize the plot's fragility and ephemerality. "Relinquish the plot," McKay writes. That is, allow the plot to

slip –
back to the unwritten:
that place where place
sleeps, where sleep itself
seeps into the landscape, having scrawled
in the pressed grass, in the bent-over reeds
its auto-erasing name.[73]

If sleep is a form of writing, it relies on disappearing ink. Because the title of Creates's installation can be read two ways – either Creates is doing the sleeping, or the places are – the photos draw attention to what the sleeping artist and the sleeping places hold in common: the absence, during sleep, of the conscious awareness of a human participant in the scene. Through the dissolving of conscious thought, Creates's identity vanishes when she falls asleep (and indeed, she is absent from the photos except as a ghostly impression), yet she is still present as the sleeper and as the artist holding the camera. Likewise, the patch of ground is always there, but it spends only a moment within the conscious gaze of the artist and the viewers of the photographs before once again going about its own business beyond the view of waking human eyes.

A final perspective on *Sleeping Places, Newfoundland 1982* comes to light through another one of Creates's photo installations, titled *Dwelling and Transience, Greater Victoria 2000*.[74] This series of fifty colour photographs portrays public signage in Victoria, British Columbia, related to the comings and goings of residents and visitors within the bustling harbour city. A sign on a lamppost, for example, reads, "TOURIST PARKING ONLY 7 A.M. TO 9 P.M., 15 MIN. MAX," and a sign directly underneath it reads, "PASSENGER ZONE, 3 MIN. MAX," a contradictory set of decrees that speaks to the complex hierarchy of land-use regulations imposed on busy city streets. Two images in particular draw the attention of anyone with sleep on their minds. A lone signpost overlooking a bare grass field with low mountains faintly visible in the distance reads, "NO PERSON MAY SLEEP OVERNIGHT IN ANY VEHICLE IN THE PARK." In a different location, on a tall lamppost in front of a short cement barrier facing the ocean, a small sign reads, "OVERNIGHT PARKING & SLEEPING PROHIBITED," with left- and right-facing arrows pointing along the length of the cement barrier.

These highly specific prohibitions, declared seemingly at random in the middle of otherwise quiet landscapes, almost comically invite a sense of mischief, especially given how easy it would be to opportunistically interpret the ambiguous wording of the signs. If "no person may sleep overnight in any vehicle in the park," can a person instead sleep in a vehicle during the day? Or for a portion of the night? What about in a tent? Can people sit in a car parked on the grass all night if they keep their eyes open? Where, exactly, are the borders of the places under the jurisdiction of these signs? How far do the left- and right-facing arrows point? By presuming to impose overly terse rules about relatively innocuous behaviour onto vaguely bordered scenic landscapes, the signs seem to parody their own authority.

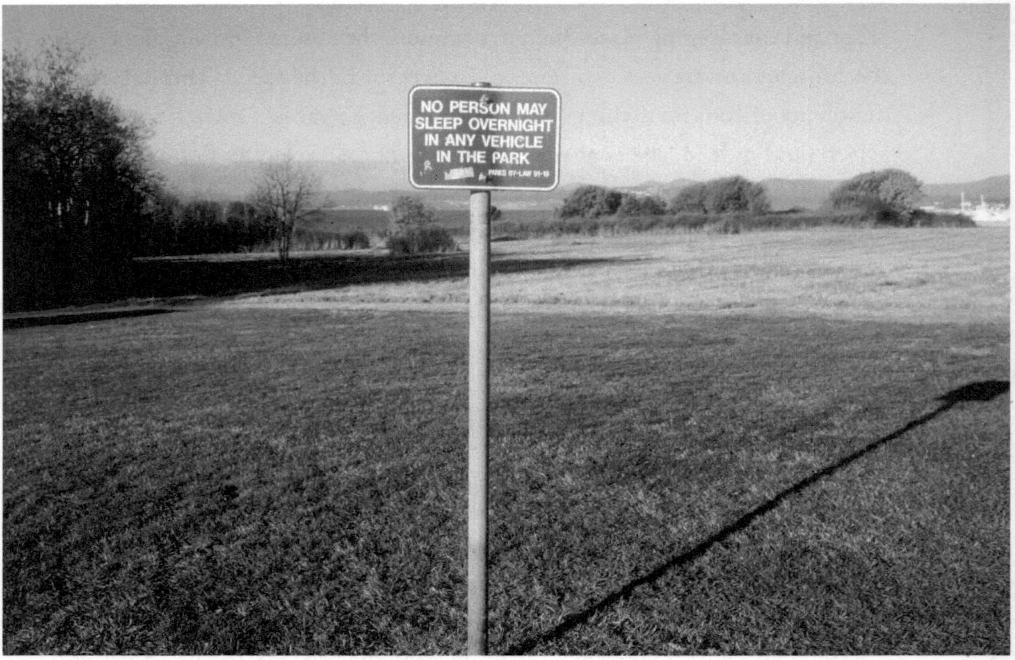

5.1 Marlene Creates, "NO PERSON MAY SLEEP OVERNIGHT IN ANY VEHICLE IN THE PARK," 2000.

Perhaps more significantly, the apparent obsession with forbidding sleep in these images forms a stark contrast to the apparently unconcerned way that Creates was able to snooze her way across the landscapes of Newfoundland eighteen years earlier. She would not be able to recreate *Sleeping Places* in the signposted areas in Victoria, even though these latter landscapes – the large, empty grassy field in particular – seem just as unlikely as the Newfoundland barrens to be bothered by the presence of a sleeper. Or rather, if she did recreate *Sleeping Places* in Victoria, the tone and connotations of the piece would be very different, casting her as a political activist and a scofflaw rather than a harmless travelling philosopher. All the rich conceptual possibilities of bringing place temporarily into existence, giving the land back to the wilderness, and imprinting one's body upon the ground are closed off when a municipal authority deems sleep to be an offence. In this way, a small signpost bearing the word "sleep" changes the very nature of the act of sleeping. The signs in Victoria were presumably erected in response to some particular perceived threat (homeless encampments, perhaps, or mildly adventurous teenagers, or tourists looking to avoid camping fees), which means that, like many prohibitions, the ban on public sleeping affects some people more than others. By converting *Sleeping Places* to *No-Sleeping Places*, as it were, the word of authority defines certain groups as troublemakers and asserts that these people can be identified as such through the act of sleeping in public view, thus recharacterizing outdoor sleep as a nefarious activity, one that is tied to the inequities of political power. The word "sleep" on a signpost can change a person's identity, and photographs of places where people have slept, might sleep, or shouldn't sleep can reveal the very different roles that sleep is made to play within the physical and cultural landscapes.

IN BED WITH OIL

In this particular stage of the Anthropocene, the conditions of sleep for many people remain highly luxurious. Memory foam mattresses, essential oil diffusers, bedtime story phone apps, central heating, air conditioning, smart light bulbs, and quiet suburbs – peculiar and flawed as these things may be – all create an infrastructure of sleep unparalleled in human history. Another thing they all have in common is a dependence on fossil fuels, as the factories, supply chains, raw materials, storefronts, and cozy bedrooms are heavily implicated in petroculture, defined by energy humanities scholar Imre Szeman as "a global society made possible by the energies afforded by burning fossil fuels."[75] For the citizens of late modernity, going to sleep at night means wrapping ourselves in the trappings of oil extraction.

In his book *Gasoline Dreams: Waking Up from Petroculture*, Hamilton-based cultural studies scholar and cartoonist Simon Orpana argues that because petroleum establishes the horizons of our collective imaginations, the difficulty of moving away from fossil fuels is as much a matter of culture as it is of politics or technology. Orpana uses sleep as a metaphor for the numbness and inattentiveness that petroculture fosters; he urges us to "wake up" by imagining new ways of living that would escape from the highways, parking lots, and inequities tied to oil.[76] "Global warming never sleeps," he says, and we, too, must figuratively stop sleeping in order to address the urgent concerns of our time. In certain cases, the trope of waking up can reflect a sleep-negative approach, casting sleep itself as a state to escape from as quickly as possible. The implications of an image, however, depend greatly on context and tone. I argued in chapter 3, in relation to the Mazda "Sleeping Roads" ad, that rather than trying to categorize every example of sleep-related discourse as being "for" or "against" good sleep, we should remain alert to figurative agendas whose representations of sleep as a symbolic figure support particular values. (We might think, for example, of the hateful political attacks on what it means to be "woke" – a notion that carries intense cultural weight but has nothing in particular to say about actual sleep.) In the case of *Gasoline Dreams*, rather than fretting over the implications of the words "wake up" for literal sleep, we can more productively approach this metaphor as an invitation to see the petroculture that we inhabit every day not as a bare and unchanging reality but as a dream world, a momentary fantasy, both beautiful and treacherous, that we can't inhabit forever.

Comprising over two hundred full-page illustrations, *Gasoline Dreams* develops much of its evocative power through visual defamiliarization. An engine gauge on the dashboard of a car is labelled "Warming," with the dial's pointer leaning heavily in that direction, and the licence plate of the car in front reads "400PPM," referring to a threshold of parts per million of carbon dioxide that was crossed in 2016, bringing our atmospheric carbon concentration to a level last seen 4 million years ago during the Pliocene era, when the world was warmer by 3 degrees Celsius.[77] Throughout the book, images of oil drip their way across the page, creeping into seemingly quotidian scenes of modern life. A child eats an ice cream bar in his mother's car, the palm of his other hand leaving oil stains on the windshield.[78] On a page about reactionary fundamentalisms, Christ's crown of thorns becomes a crown of leaking oil pipelines.[79] The otherwise featureless monolith from the movie *2001: A Space Odyssey*,[80] surrounded by early hominids about to grasp the power of technology, gains a slot that serves as a holster for a gas pump nozzle.[81] These images call upon us to see the familiar objects and practices of everyday life, as well as the iconography and media that surround us, in a strange new light, where they become the dreamy manifestations of a petroleum-driven world. Most notably of all, each illustration is rendered entirely in dirty smudges and splatters of black ink, as though the entire text, like the petroculture from which it comes, has been given its form through the use of oil.

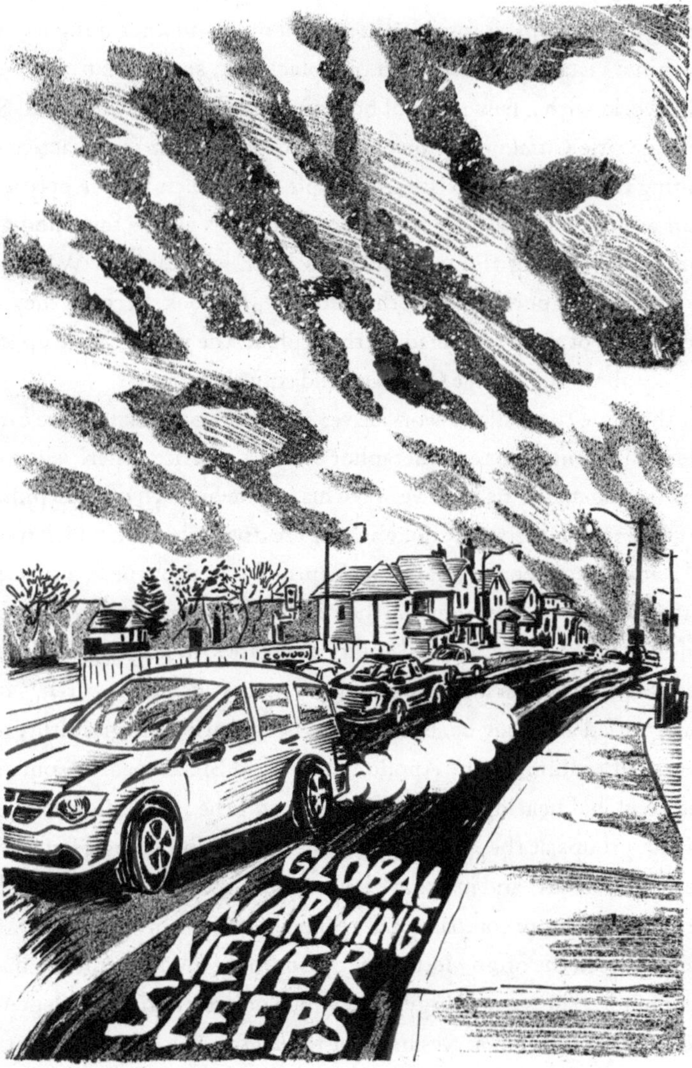

5.2 Simon Orpana, *Gasoline Dreams: Waking Up from Petroculture* (2021), 47.

These pages imply that until we do the demanding work of fully imagining a world beyond fossil fuels, there is no ready vantage point that can enable us to view petroculture from the "outside." When toxic clouds of pollution spell out the enormous words "Wake up," and when the line "Global warming never sleeps" is scrawled in asphalt on a landscape designed for cars, all within a vista illustrated with oily black ink, such a text requires us to see the world with a new sense of both intimacy and irony. As with *Sleeping Places*, the title *Gasoline Dreams* turns two ways. Who is the active subject dreaming the world into existence: people or petroleum? The petrocultural terrain within which we live is rendered here as a visible force and a call to action rather than as an inert backdrop or an inevitability. When readers step outside after putting down their copy of the book, perhaps they will see the metaphor of sleep inscribed on the asphalt, the words "wake up" written in the sky above the Dodge Caravans and suburban homes.

At the same time, such a work leaves room for us to ask how we can imagine sleep differently, not as a metaphor but as a practice. There is a real sense in which sleep makes us who we are. This is true for each of us as individuals since the forms of memory, thought, and creativity through which we understand ourselves depend crucially on sleep, and it is also true at a species level. Humans appear to be unique in the high proportion of REM sleep that we attain each night, and our social ability to create safe sleeping conditions has helped us to survive in hazardous environments across the earth.[82] Human sleep, as varied as it may be, is linked to the invention of agriculture and the discovery of radium, to the Apollo rockets and Shakespeare's sonnets. It is linked to global heating, mass extinction, and the methodical exploitation of certain groups at the hands of others. The creative energies of sleep have made us who we are, and just maybe, we can use these energies to build a new, more equitable, more compassionate home in the Anthropocene.

Oil is indeed the often hidden energy source of modern culture, but sleep, too, is a hidden source of energy upon which our cultural world depends. We may deplete our sleep reserves in order to fuel social acceleration, but we can also find within sleep a fount of alternative inspiration. What might sleep look like in a world no longer tied to the narratives and supply chains built on oil? As the neoliberal vision of self-reliance runs up against the need for collective ecological action, how will we negotiate sleep as a practice that is at once social and individual? How can we learn to invent, read, and share good sleep amidst the anxieties of ecological collapse? If our collective response to the climate crisis will be judged by how we mitigate its terrible inequities, how might we come to understand equitable access to good sleep as a measure of climate justice? Orpana writes that "we can't know ahead of time what life under a different energy system will look or feel like. It will surely bring new relationships, opportunities and struggles."[83] The changeability of our future relationship with sleep is all the more reason to continue approaching such questions with thoughtfulness, curiosity, and hope long after you close the pages of his book or this one.

The conditions of sleep are not separate from waking life, and the concerns that characterize the waking world – love, pleasure, safety, meaningful work, precarity, loss, and grief – forever intertwine with the ways that we sleep or fail to sleep. If we want to create good conditions for sleep, we should work toward energy transition, reconciliation, good working conditions, social safety nets, and other ways of fostering equity for everyone. We should fight climate change like our very bedrooms depend on it, which they do. From blankets and pillows to the dreams that we have on them, the way that we sleep will undergo great transformations in the coming years. There is no opting out of the problem of sleeping on a precarious, damaged, warming planet, but the decisions that we make about confronting ecological collapse will help to shape what sleep in the Anthropocene looks like, both in its inequities and troubles and in its enchantment and hope.

CONCLUSION

The Work of Sleep

IN UNTANGLING THE CULTURAL MEANINGS of sleep, my focus in this book has not been to provide you with practical tips to improve your own literal sleep. Luckily, however, critical sleep studies does have the benefit of helping us to promote good slumber. Indeed, it would be a sad mistake to focus so hard on sleep as a cultural figure that we forget to teach one another to sleep well. Arguing that "justice is good for your sleep," philosopher Benjamin Hale and public health scholar Lauren Hale write that "a measure of the just society is the degree to which its citizens are sleeping well and are healthy."[1] Bringing about a decent and equitable society requires us to sleep with care as well as to read sleep with care.

Self-help books will tell you to improve your sleep by lowering your room temperature, going to bed late enough that you actually feel sleepy, setting a consistent morning alarm, and practising mindfulness techniques. These tips can be truly useful, and if you want to gain better control over your sleep, I suggest reading a book such as Gregg D. Jacobs's *Say Good Night to Insomnia* or W. Chris Winter's *The Sleep Solution* or talking to your doctor about behavioural modification therapy. However, individual behaviour can only go so far in addressing structural problems, and you may have to endure some frustration when you are told, as Jacobs says, that "the key to conquering insomnia resides within you."[2] After all, the distinction between insomnia – the personal inability to sleep well – and sleep deprivation imposed by external factors such as overwork or stressful caregiving is not always clear-cut. This is just one reason that fostering better sleep for everyone depends on cultural changes. As journalist Anna North writes, "while there are steps people can take in their own lives to address insomnia, sleep deprivation isn't just a personal problem; it's also a social one."[3] She calls for shorter working hours, better pay, and comprehensive health care for all. Author and public health scholar James Hamblin similarly argues that "the most effective way to improve sleep is to ensure that people have a calm and quiet place to rest each night, free of concerns about basic needs such as food security."[4] We must remember these arguments when we are presented with solutions or warnings that see sleep purely at the level of the individual consumer or psychological subject. Sleep is a matter of equity, culture, and power, and by rethinking sleep, we can imagine a better, more equitable society.

Recognizing the cultural nature of sleep can inspire us to champion good slumber in unexpected ways. For instance, labour unions can advocate powerfully for living wages and equitable protection from overwork. People who believed in the power of unions in the nineteenth century fought to banish the ten-hour work day and the six-day work week, granting people "eight hours for work, eight hours for sleep, eight hours for what we will."[5] In a twenty-first-century world of continuous digital connection, fast turnaround times, and gig labour, reawakening the nineteenth-century call for protected hours of sleep is crucially important, whether this initiative takes the form of policies that guarantee the "right to disconnect," laws that classify gig workers as employees with access to benefits, or the protection of guaranteed public services and minimum incomes.[6]

Moreover, the fostering of good sleep must be based on a commitment to gender equity and anti-racism. As argued by Tricia Hersey with regard to her work at the Nap Ministry, sleep and resting can serve as radical anti-racist acts in the context of capitalism, grind culture, and white supremacy. Speaking to the experience of Black people in the United States in particular, she argues that "our lack of resting has stolen our imagination and our ability to be inventive and subversive and to imagine and to have hope. And to me, that's true oppression … If you can't imagine how you could subversively and flexibly rest your eyes for 10 minutes, how could we ever imagine a world without police? How do we imagine a world without climate change? … A new world is possible, but it's not going to come from exhaustion."[7] Hersey's approach sees sleep as an initiative toward justice, creativity, and fuller humanity. This undertaking can create a virtuous circle, where the commitment to an activist mindset creates space for more restful sleep and where sleep itself serves an activist function by resisting legacies of inequity and harm. As Hersey is well aware, the penalties for frequent napping and resting can be severe for people who barely get by on hourly wages.[8] Consequently, fostering sleep as activism must work in concert with the initiatives above, such as guaranteed incomes and, as mentioned in the previous chapter, strong action toward climate justice.

As we work toward better sleep by lowering our thermostats and demanding better social safety nets, however, let us remember that sleeping better does not always have to be the goal. Another worthy aspiration is to learn to forgive ourselves, and each other, for flawed sleep. Lying awake sometimes is a very human thing to do, and sleeplessness does not always have to be pathologized or targeted for relentless self-improvement. Sometimes, for health reasons or otherwise, good sleep is simply impossible, and there are times when we may need to accept lousy sleep as a normal part of life, like rainy weather. On those nights, maybe the best sleep is the one you can get – and if that sleep leaves much to be desired, you are certainly in good company. One of the paradoxes of insomnia is the sense in which your solitary vigil in the lonely hours of the night means that you truly belong to your social world.

Whether we are hoping to sleep better or are learning to live with the sleep that we've got, critical sleep studies teaches us how to see sleep not just as an individual matter but also as a cultural one. A key message of this book has been that if we want to understand the seemingly innocent and private practice of slumber as a site of cultural meaning and power, we need to develop a critical literacy of sleep and imagination; we need to be careful readers of the sleep socialization stories that surround us all. The critical study of sleep can challenge and expand the conceptual building blocks through which we see the world, an exercise that is aesthetic and shocking, beautiful and dangerous, solitary and social – one that both engages with and goes beyond politics by embracing the human realities of ambiguity and feeling.

Such an approach can also serve as a vital method for upholding the importance of the humanities in investigating concerns that are usually assumed to belong to the realms of science, technology, and consumer capitalism. With regard to sleep, the humanities will do what they do best: teach us how to engage in critical questioning of loud authorities and silent assumptions. They will identify how cultural forms of power influence our perceptions of value. They will reveal technological and scientific approaches to sleep for what they are: inspired paths of discovery that do not simply make the truth about sleep visible but also shape and construct the very meaning of sleep in ways that reinforce the centrality of technology to human existence. Through the humanities, we can step back from these visions of sleep with irony, humour, and incisiveness. When a large societal problem arises, sleep-related or otherwise, one of our goals should be to foster a public sphere where people do not instinctively say, "Maybe there is a new app and tracking device that can solve this problem," but instead ask, "How can we reframe this problem and challenge it at an imaginative and structural level?" Critical sleep studies gives us the tools to engage in this kind of intervention, and the skills that emerge from literary analysis and cultural studies are key because they allow us to see seemingly mundane visions of sleep through fresh eyes. Through literary works and other thoughtful texts, we can both learn and unlearn how to imagine sleep.

Sleep has intrinsic value and should not be a form of work, something we do purely to enhance frantic productivity. However, when we are awake, we can do good work with regard to the meanings and conditions of sleep. To this end, I have provided a brief appendix with sample exercises. Whether you approach these exercises as an instructor, a student, a reader, an insomniac, or a champion sleeper, I hope you find them useful for reimagining sleep in a restless world. If you are willing to undertake further adventures in critical sleep studies, I would love to hear about them. Send me an email so that I can learn to see sleep through your eyes.

In Canada and elsewhere, the cultural and literary politics of sleep will extend far beyond the texts and practices that I have discussed in this book, which is part of the point. Learning to read sleep cannot just be a matter of examining certain texts in great detail; rather, we need to foster the critical discernment and flexibility of mind that will allow us to respond wisely and thoughtfully to those texts and practices that we have not yet seen. The project of untangling sleep will require ongoing attention to diverse voices from across the full spectrum of power and disempowerment. Much like water or medicine, sleep is a universal need whose allocation is tied to unequal forms of privilege. For this reason, sleep cannot so easily be separated from the context of ideological priorities and from the forms of manipulation that make the experience of sleep and sleeplessness different for diverse groups of people. Sleep is crucial, contested, enchanting, and inequitable, and it increasingly finds itself in the public spotlight in a way that will benefit greatly from the forms of critical literacy fostered within the humanities. A literary vision of slumber is in a unique position to engage with sleep as both aesthetics and politics, as both practice and representation. Every sleep tells a story, and by learning to read with care, we can help each other to rest a little easier.

APPENDIX

Your Sleep Assignment

These suggested assignments offer some ideas for building a critical literacy of sleep in and beyond the classroom. If you are an instructor, feel free to use or adapt these ideas in any way that you like. Please acknowledge this book as the source of the exercises, and send me an email (phuebener@athabascau.ca) if you find them useful.

SLEEP REFLECTIONS

1 Engage with your own personal sleep in a way that is different from your usual routine. For example, you might turn off your alarm, adopt a nocturnal lifestyle, sleep in a hammock, sleep on a memory foam pillow, start using a bedtime phone app, stop using a bedtime phone app, take a nap on a riverbank, sleep according to a self-help book, sleep alone, sleep with others, or recall how your sleeping habits changed during the Covid-19 pandemic. Develop a critical analysis of your sleep experience, including your successes, your frustrations, and the implications of your cultural surroundings for your sleep. You may also consider how you could extend this kind of activity to make it an ongoing reflection.

2 If you live in Canada or in another place that has colonized Indigenous land, consider your own relationship with sleep in terms of traditional territory. For example, how might you trace the history and values of your cultural world by considering

your sleep practices on this land? Are you sleeping in a place where someone else's sleep has been displaced? In what sense has your sleep been colonized or decolonized? How might you approach the process of reconciliation by considering the value and inequities of sleep? The Canadian Association of University Teachers has published a *Guide to Acknowledging First Peoples and Traditional Territory* that may be useful as a starting point. For example, Edmonton is located on Treaty 6 territory, Calgary is on Treaty 7 territory, Ottawa is on the unceded territory of the Algonquin Anishnaabeg People, and Vancouver is on the unceded territory of the Coast Salish Peoples. Develop a critical personal reflection on your position, with reference to selected readings.

3 Find a "text" of your own choosing – perhaps an advertisement, a speech, an app, a map, a legal code, a television show, a movie, a photograph, a song, a poem, an activity, a consumer product, some other cultural object, or something from your ecosystem – and develop an analysis of how this text conceives of sleep. You might ask these questions or others: How does the text develop meaning through sleep? How does it link sleep with other concerns? What assumptions about sleep does it contain or resist? Does it portray sleep as a literal act or as a symbolic figure, and to what end? Whose sleep matters in this text? If sleep is not represented explicitly, how does it arise implicitly? For ideas, you can refer to work related to critical sleep studies, such as Simon J. Williams's *The Politics of Sleep*, Benjamin Reiss's *Wild Nights*, Sarah Sharma's *In the Meantime*, and articles by Sara Arber, Diletta De Cristofaro, and other scholars included in the bibliography.

4 Analyze the representation of sleep in one or more literary texts, such as Sandra Huber's *Assembling the Morrow*, Tracey Lindberg's *Birdie*, Suzette Mayr's *The Sleeping Car Porter*, Nino Ricci's *Sleep*, Michael Ondaatje's *In the Skin of a Lion*, David Chariandy's *Brother*, Sylvia Legris's *Nerve Squall*, Ottessa Moshfegh's *My Year of Rest and Relaxation*, Adrian Barnes's *Nod*, Kenneth Calhoun's

Black Moon, Karen Thompson Walker's *The Dreamers*, or others. Refer to existing criticism and selected readings in critical sleep studies, such as those included in the bibliography.

5 Create a series of social media posts that apply some of the concepts raised in critical sleep studies. Perhaps you will post some comments on a new book about sleep, review a movie using a critical sleep studies perspective, or create a blog where you analyze the cultural politics of government policy announcements with regard to sleep. If you find a package of herbal tea with an illustration of a sleeping teddy bear, you might post a photo of the package alongside an analysis of the illustration. Enrich your discussion by considering how you might extend or challenge the ideas that have been raised by scholars in critical sleep studies.

NOTES

ACKNOWLEDGMENTS

1 Younging, *Elements of Indigenous Style*, 15.

INTRODUCTION

1 CBC *News*, "30% of Canadian Men."

2 See, for instance, Huber, *Assembling the Morrow*, 24. I, too, was once surprised after an EEG reported that I had slept more deeply than I thought.

3 Ibid, 10. The actual study in question is Nobili et al., "Local Aspects of Sleep."

4 Augustine, *Confessions*, bk 11, ch. 14. Although Augustine does not seem to worry overmuch about how to define sleep, his dismay about the lustfulness of his dreams results in a crisis of identity. "And yet there is so much difference betwixt myself and myself," he writes, "within that moment wherein I pass from waking to sleeping, or return from sleeping to waking!" (bk 10, ch. 30).

5 On the problems with sleep associated with modernity, see for example, Reiss, *Wild Nights*, 15; and Lockley and Foster, *Sleep*, 2.

6 Lockley and Foster, *Sleep*, 2. When using the word "we," Lockley and Foster are focusing mainly on people in Britain and other industrialized nations.

7 Chaput, Wong, and Michaud, "Duration and Quality."

8 MacDonald, "Canadians."

9 One contrarian view comes from psychophysiologist Jim Horne, who argues that "sleep debt is overstated, as the great majority of us have sufficient sleep, especially as our 7-hour average sleep has changed little over the last century." Horne, *Sleeplessness*, preface. Another study that "challenge[s] the claim of increasingly sleep-deprived societies" is Bin, Marshall, and Glozier, "Sleeping at the Limits," 826, which suggests that the average sleep quantity in industrialized countries may actually be *increasing*, although, as with most sleep surveys, the data have significant limitations. For additional discussion of the "sleep crisis thesis," see Greaney, *Sleep and the Novel*, ch. 6. Important work on the cultural implications of these issues is being done by the research group Writing the Sleep Crisis, led by Diletta De Cristofaro.

10 Rao et al., "Informing Sleep Policy," 530.

11 For Ekirch's insights, see his book *At Day's Close*. For examples of responses and rebuttals to the segmented sleep theory, see Reiss's discussion in *Wild Nights*, 34ff. Ekirch himself says that he has seen no reason to adopt segmented sleep in

his own life, adding that "at no time in history have conditions for human slumber been better than today." Quoted in Thompson, "Can Medieval Sleeping?"

12 Reiss, *Wild Nights*, 36.

13 Problems with preindustrial sleep included not only insect pests but also nighttime crime, fires, leaky roofs, and excessive heat and cold. See Thompson, "Can Medieval Sleeping?"

14 See, for example, Lockley and Russell, *Sleep*, ch. 7, or any number of reader-friendly sources, such as Cleveland Clinic, "Here's What Happens"; Centers for Disease Control and Prevention, "Sleep and Chronic Disease"; Winter, *Sleep Solution*, ch. 1; as well as other sources cited below. For an example of a government publication discussing sleep and health in Canada, see Chaput, Wong, and Michaud, "Duration and Quality." Much like the question of whether there really is a modern sleep crisis, the health consequences of sleep loss are also subject to some debate, the argument being that "adverse health effects are often overstated." Horne, *Sleeplessness*, ch. 14. Cautious writers tend to emphasize that sleep loss and poor health are "linked" or "associated," but many publications assert direct causal effects. As a nonscientist, my overall impression from the literature is that although sorting out correlation and causation is a difficult process, chronic sleep loss is indeed very unhealthy.

15 Walker, *Why We Sleep*, 132. Walker's bestselling book has attracted some degree of controversy over the accuracy of its specific claims about sleep science. At the very least, the book is important as a high-profile example of public discourse and anxiety around sleep.

16 Ibid., ch. 8.

17 On blue-light-blocking glasses, see Yousef, "There's No Evidence." On power naps, see for example, my discussion of Nap It Up in chapter 1. On naps and Alzheimer's, see Devlin, "Long Naps." On sleeping during pregnancy, see Ross-White, "Sleeping on Your Back." On worrying about insomnia, see CBC *News*, "Poor Quality, Short Sleep." This is not even to speak of the terrifying and ever-shifting set of instructions given to new parents about the countless, often expensive ways that they must regulate the conditions of their baby's sleep to keep it from dying. See, for example, Donkin, "Unsafe Sleep."

18 Lee, "Sleep Deprivation."

19 Athabasca University, "Mothers Who Don't." In responding to stories that appear to blame mothers for sleep loss, we can turn to Sara Arber's research group, which has found that when women lose sleep due to behaviours such as worrying, their lack of sleep is often portrayed as an individual psychological problem rather than an effect of socially prescribed gender roles that require emotional labour. Arber, Meadows, and Venn, "Sleep and Society," 241. Here, Arber's group also notes that socio-economic disadvantages tend to create more sleep problems for women.

20 Reiss, *Wild Nights*, 5 (quote), 23.

21 Arber, Meadows, and Venn, "Sleep and Society," 231.

22 McKinnon, "Feminist Philosopher."
23 Ortiz-Ospina, "How Do People?"
24 Crary, *24/7*, 11.
25 Greaney, *Sleep and the Novel*, ch. 1.
26 Carson, "Every Exit," 19.
27 In producing the term "sleep socialization stories," I am drawing from my earlier work on what I have called "time socialization stories." See, for example, Huebener, *Nature's Broken Clocks*, 2.
28 Greaney argues that "one of the most notable achievements of work in the field of critical sleep studies has been to dispel … the 'Myth of Natural Sleep.'" Greaney, *Sleep and the Novel*, ch. 6, citing science and technology scholar Matthew J. Wolf-Meyer.
29 Greaney, *Sleep and the Novel*, ch. 1.
30 Reiss, *Wild Nights*, 12 (quote), 61.
31 Ibid., 122.
32 Arber, Meadows, and Venn, "Sleep and Society," 224, original emphasis.
33 Ibid., 223.
34 Ibid., 235, 234; see also esp. 242. Studies on these concerns have often been based in the United States or (as with Arber and her collaborators) in the United Kingdom. Anthropologist Carol M. Worthman, who has undertaken cross-cultural sleep studies, finds that sleep practices in general are "largely culturally determined, and that cultural models and morals infuse sleep behavior, settings, and sensibilities." Worthman, "Developmental Cultural Ecology," 189.
35 Crary, *24/7*, 10.
36 When commentators warn, for example, that the metaverse – a global virtual reality meeting place – is destined "to mine every human interaction in the world for data that can then be monetized," we would do well to consider the implications for sleep. Rose, "Zuckerberg's Meta Endgame."
37 Berg and Seeber, *Slow Professor*, 29.
38 Hersey, *Rest Is Resistance*, 33, 7.
39 Ibid., 8.
40 Ibid., 16.
41 Williams, *Politics of Sleep*, introduction.
42 Ibid.
43 Ibid.
44 Hersey, *Rest Is Resistance*, 25.
45 De Cristofaro and Chiodo, "Quantified Sleep," 183.
46 Ibid., 183, 178, 177.
47 Hinds, *Cultural History*, 5.
48 Ermine, "Aboriginal Epistemology," 108–9.
49 Scrivner, "That Sweet Secession," 269.
50 Ibid., 276.
51 G.A. Sullivan Jr, *Sleep, Romance*, 1.

52 Reiss, *Wild Nights*, 16.
53 Ibid., 215.
54 Heyes, "We're Not Dreamers." As of this writing, Heyes is developing "the first feminist philosophy of sleep." Since this project has not yet been published, I have cited the abstract from one of Heyes's public lectures.
55 Greaney, *Sleep and the Novel*, chs 1 and 7, original emphasis.
56 Ibid., ch. 7.

CHAPTER ONE

1 The percentage of people in Canada who experience trouble sleeping is difficult to measure, with different survey methodologies giving different results. In a 2020 survey conducted by Statistics Canada, "half of respondents reported trouble going to sleep or staying asleep sometimes, most of the time or all the time," but "the majority of Canadian adults obtained adequate sleep." Wang et al., "Sleep Behaviours." The *Globe and Mail* reported in 2022 that "experts from the Royal Ottawa Institute of Mental Health Research estimate that half the population in Canada now struggles with some sort of sleep-related problem." MacDonald, "Canadians." However, I am unable to locate such a statement from the institute, and even if the claim is true, many of these sleep problems may be mild. On the inequitable distribution of sleep loss, see Chaput et al., "Prevalence of Insomnia." See also the work of Sara Arber and her collaborators in the United Kingdom, who have found that sleep problems tend to be linked to gender, age, social class, and income. Arber, Meadows, and Venn, "Sleep and Society."
2 Wang et al., "Sleep Behaviours."
3 Chaput et al., "Prevalence of Insomnia."
4 Indra Narang, quoted in McCue, "Lack of Sleep." Additional commentary on sleep in children is available in MacDonald, "Canadians."
5 MacDonald, "Canadians"; McCue, "Lack of Sleep."
6 Wang et al., "Sleep Behaviours."
7 Chaput et al., "Prevalence of Insomnia."
8 This figure comes from ibid. As with most sleep surveys, interpretive caution is advisable. The authors note a problem, for example, with "different definitions of insomnia in the literature."
9 Winter, *Sleep Solution*, 148.
10 Ibid., 150.
11 Statistics Canada, "Table 45-10-0014-01."
12 Chaput, Wong, and Michaud, "Duration and Quality."
13 CBC *News*, "New UVic Research." The information in the following sentence also comes from this report.
14 Wible, "What I've Learned."
15 Ibid.

16 For detailed discussions of time use as it relates to occupations such as taxi driving and hotel housekeeping, see Sharma, *In the Meantime*.
17 Quoted in Larsen, "Former Canucks." For commentary on the broader use of Ambien in the National Hockey League, including the overdose death of New York Rangers forward Derek Boogaard, see Dater, "Ambien Use."
18 Statistics Canada, "Table 45-10-0014-01." Again, this kind of discrepancy is difficult to measure with certainty.
19 The information here and in the next few sentences is from Hounsell, "1 in 4 Seniors."
20 For example, both Chaput et al., "Prevalence of Insomnia," and Chaput, Wong, and Michaud, "Duration and Quality," draw their data from the Canadian Health Measures Survey, in which, as these studies explain, "residents of First Nations Reserves or other Aboriginal settlements, institutions and some remote regions, and full-time members of the Canadian Forces were excluded."
21 Daschuk, *Clearing the Plains*, 176.
22 Ibid.
23 For an account of this event, including an audio interview with witness Tatjana Shawanamash-Ignace, see Turner, "Images of Security."
24 Waterfield, "Strong Rebuke."
25 Whyte, "Indigenous Climate Change," 154.
26 Ibid.
27 Watt-Cloutier, *Right to Be Cold*, ch. 6.
28 Ibid.
29 Traill, *Backwoods of Canada*, letter 11.
30 Moodie, *Roughing It*, ch. 15.
31 Ibid., ch. 13.
32 Ibid., ch. 22.
33 Ibid., ch. 4.
34 Traill, *Backwoods of Canada*, letter 13.
35 T. Wong, *Dear Scarlet*, 45, 89.
36 Ibid., 73.
37 Ibid., 59–60.
38 See, for example, Grandner et al., "Who Gets the Best Sleep?" which links lower socio-economic status with greater sleep disturbances.
39 Patten, *Tower 25*, 15.
40 Ibid., 19, 17.
41 Ibid., 22.
42 Ibid., 21.
43 Ibid., 28.
44 Ibid., 69.
45 Ibid., 107–11.
46 Ibid., 126.

47 The problem of being denied the dignity of sleep can also resonate among migrants who fear deportation. A recent study in Toronto of Mexican migrants with precarious status relates the story of Rebeca, a mother of two children from Mexico City who is working at a cleaning job but has overstayed her visitor's visa. Describing the painful uncertainty of this experience, Rebeca speaks of "the inability to do anything, not even buy a bed because you don't know if you are leaving the next day." Quoted in Villegas, "I can't even," 283.
48 The details and quotations in this paragraph come from Sharma, *In the Meantime*, 142–3, original emphasis.
49 Ibid., 144.
50 Sharkey, "Do Libraries?"
51 Nap It Up, "Services."
52 Sharma makes a similar observation when she notes that openly sleeping in public – on a Tokyo subway car, for example, or in an airport sleep pod – tends to be permitted when the sleeper is a business worker taking a power nap. In these cases, "a dark business suit absolves a sleepyhead from regulation." Sharma, *In the Meantime*, 48.
53 Centre for Sleep and Human Performance, "About."
54 CTV *News*, "Canada's First Napping."
55 Regarding Trudeau's famous comment about the decriminalization of private homosexual acts in 1967, the CBC notes that "Trudeau may have made the 'bedrooms of the nation' phrase famous but it was actually coined by The Globe and Mail's Martin O'Malley. Trudeau thanked O'Malley for the quotation." CBC, "Trudeau."
56 *Daily Hive*, "Capture Photography."
57 Harris, "By Covering Up."
58 Wall, "Statement on Removal."
59 Ibid.
60 Heard, "Vancouver Billboards."
61 Wall, "Statement on Removal."
62 For Niro's statement of identity, see "Artist Statements," in Mockler et al., *Watch Your Head*.
63 Ermine, "Aboriginal Epistemology," 108–9.
64 Reiss, *Wild Nights*, 25.
65 Simpson, "Stories, Dreams, and Ceremonies."
66 @netflix, "Sleep is my greatest enemy."
67 Sleep Country Canada, "About Us."
68 Arber, Meadows, and Venn, "Sleep and Society," 229.
69 Sleep Country Canada, "What Keeps You Awake?"
70 On personal habits and anxieties that contribute to insomnia, see for example, Winter, *Sleep Solution*. On systemic factors behind sleep loss, see Arber, Meadows, and Venn, "Sleep and Society."
71 Sleep Country Canada, "Turn off the Lights."

72 *The Onion*, "Weighted Blanket Sure to Succeed."
73 Sleep Country Canada, "#SleepIsForTheStrong."
74 Ibid., descriptive text accompanying the YouTube ad.
75 Hinds, *Cultural History*, 5.
76 In addition to relying on ecologically costly global supply chains – Bloom, for instance, is manufactured in China and then shipped overseas – the mattress-in-a-box industry at large has been training the public to see mattresses as disposable goods. Customers can typically return their mattress for a full refund even several months after buying it – which they often do, not having tried it beforehand – yet mattresses are notoriously poor candidates for recycling, causing what the *Guardian* calls "a global environmental nightmare." Kale, "Mattress Landfill Crisis." In an unusual move for online sales, Sleep Country does not offer refunds on Bloom mattresses (only store credit), and they claim to reuse or recycle returned mattresses. By contrast, consider the Haven mattress company, whose products are made in Canada from "vegan plant-based foams" using "soy based gel" as part of a commitment to the environment. Haven Sleep Company, "Common Mattress Questions." These odd food-like ingredients could easily be satirized, yet the notion that such bedding is considered a niche product emphasizes that the use of synthetic, sometimes toxic materials and ecologically costly supply chains is assumed to be the norm. The study of how contemporary bedding products illuminate cultural forms of value could extend far beyond these examples.
77 Arber, Meadows, and Venn, "Sleep and Society," 228–9.
78 Rosa, *Social Acceleration*, 87.
79 Sharma, *In the Meantime*, 106.
80 Sleep Country Canada, "Sleep Is the Fuel" (11 July 2020); Sleep Country Canada, "Sleep Is the Fuel" (17 July 2020); Sleep Country Canada, "To Power Your Day."
81 De Cristofaro and Chiodo, "Quantified Sleep," 191.
82 Ibid., 185.
83 Sleep Country Canada, "Sleep Is the Fuel" (17 July 2020).
84 Stern, "College Mantra."
85 The gendered nuances of the maxim "sleep is for the weak" are made more complex when the phrase is used as an expression of hypermasculine strength. Vancouver folk-punk band The Dreadnoughts, for instance, released a song called "Sleep Is for the Weak" on their 2010 album *Polka's Not Dead*. The song exudes a performative masculinity in its celebration of alcohol-fuelled, sleepless, late-night hijinks, with lyrics that are screamed and growled as much as they are sung: "You'll greet the sun with bottles high ... Up into the highest peak / Sleep is for the weak." The Swedish metal band DEMOTIONAL also uses the phrase as a song title. One might say that such songs both celebrate and parody the performance of masculine strength. Interestingly, the phrase is used here to reject, not endorse, the culture of productivity, thus subverting the culture of

overwork in a way that most uses of the maxim do not. However, this subversion is accomplished through brutally masculine screamed lyrics. An implication is that men can declare that sleep is for the weak so that they can party into the night, whereas women must declare that sleep is for the weak in order to endure the exhaustion of parenting. This reading of the music may depend on the degree of irony one perceives in the band's performance.

86 Hersey, *Rest Is Resistance*, 94, 150. For commentary on the notion of resilience specifically, see for instance, the discussion of mandatory resilience among exhausted social workers, a situation that embodies "the neoliberal trend of downloading responsibility onto individuals," in Zhou and Coxson, "'Resilient' Social Workers," 64.

87 In a motivational speech that became a viral video, actor and politician Arnold Schwarzenegger tells his audience that anyone can achieve greatness if they fully dedicate their time to their goals. Anyone who is indulgent enough to sleep more than six hours a night, he says, needs to "just sleep faster." See "Arnold Schwarzenegger 2018."

88 See Fagan, "Bizarre Social History."

CHAPTER TWO

1 Heyes, "Anaesthetics of Existence," 276.

2 Reiss, *Wild Nights*, 217.

3 Ibid., 219, original emphasis.

4 Greaney, *Sleep and the Novel*, ch. 5.

5 Ibid.

6 Ibid., original emphasis.

7 Ricoeur, *Time and Narrative*, vol. 3, 246.

8 Ibid., vol. 1, 3.

9 For commentary on the Lunesta moth and the ethics of sleep aid drug ads, see Aubrey, "Drug Ads."

10 rawlings, *Wide Slumber*, 24.

11 Ibid., 42.

12 Ibid., 98, 98, 100.

13 Groeneveld, "Unsettling the Environment," 149.

14 Ibid., 142. Scholar Erin Gray, who examines *Wide Slumber* in the context of contemporary Canadian feminist poetics, also finds that by dismantling the objective language of science and focusing on bodily experience, the poem serves as a feminist refusal of patriarchal discourse. Gray, "Good Sentences."

15 On the problem of men sexually assaulting women who are asleep, see Moore, "Sexual Assault."

16 Bell, "Trippy State."

17 Domanski, "Hypnagogia," 20–1.

18 Atwood, "Variation," 77.

19 The poem does not specify the genders of the speaker and the person being addressed. Both Jill Hufnagel and Heather Heckman-McKenna refer to the speaker as female and assert that the addressee is male, which is reasonable in the context of Atwood's body of work about gender politics from this time period and is consistent with the poem's use of certain symbols and tropes. I am following this convention out of consistency rather than certainty. Hufnagel, "Atwood's Variation"; Heckman-McKenna, "Redefining Love."
20 Hufnagel, "Atwood's Variation," 188.
21 Ibid., 189.
22 The poetry quotation is from Atwood, "Variation," 77. The assertion by Hufnagel is based on her comments in "Atwood's Variation," 188.
23 Heckman-McKenna, "Redefining Love," 93.
24 Cohen, "Two Went to Sleep," 25.
25 Brand, *Thirsty*, 63.
26 Vizenor, *Manifest Manners*, vii.
27 Ipellie, "Waking Up," 294–6.
28 Deerchild, "bread crumbs," 568–9.
29 Deerchild, "mama making moccasins," 566.
30 Ibid., 565.
31 Belleau, "Sunday," 604.
32 McAdam, "Hot Women," 25.
33 Shepherd, "Crescent," 92.
34 Kulchyski, *Aboriginal Rights*, 165, quoted as an epigraph in ibid. with the line breaks shown here.
35 The quoted lines in this paragraph are from Shepherd, "Cultural Darwinism," 26.
36 J. Butler, *Magnetic North*, "The Journey."
37 Ibid.
38 Ibid., "Ornithomancy."
39 Ibid., "Night."
40 Ibid.
41 Williams, *Politics of Sleep*, ch. 5.
42 See Crary, *24/7*, 1; and Randall, *Dreamland*, 151.
43 Randall, *Dreamland*, 152.
44 On Vietnam and post-traumatic stress disorder, see Nudelman, *Fighting Sleep*, 4. On Afghanistan and Iraq, see Amin et al., "War-Related Illness," 156.
45 Findley, *Wars*, 184.
46 Brand, *Inventory*, 83.
47 The biographical details in this section come from Hertwig, "Home from the War."
48 Ibid.
49 Moncur, "I Almost Died."
50 Hertwig, *Slow War*, 69.
51 Ibid., 58.

52 Ibid., 19.
53 Ibid., 20.
54 Ibid.
55 Ibid., 27.
56 Ibid., 28.
57 Marsh, "In Flanders Fields."
58 McCrae, "In Flanders Fields."
59 Sugars, *Canadian Gothic*, 2.
60 Holmes, "'In Flanders Fields,'" 21; McCutcheon, "'Come on back,'" 771.
61 McCutcheon, "'Come on back,'" 771.
62 Hertwig, *Slow War*, 101–2.
63 McGregor, "'Between history,'" 3.
64 Williams, *Politics of Sleep*, introduction.

CHAPTER THREE

1 Greaney, *Sleep and the Novel*, ch. 1.
2 Maracle, *Daughters Are Forever*, 19. Maracle is a member of the Sto:lo First Nation.
3 E. Robinson, *Monkey Beach*, 139. Robinson is a member of the Haisla and Heiltsuk First Nations.
4 Re:Searching for LGBTQ2S+ Health, "Two-Spirit Community."
5 Whitehead, *Jonny Appleseed*, ch. 45.
6 Ibid., ch. 29.
7 Ibid., ch. 26.
8 Ibid., ch. 28.
9 Ibid., ch. 41.
10 Ibid.
11 Ibid., ch. 35.
12 Ibid., ch. 21.
13 Cooper, "Future Perfect," 491.
14 Whitehead, *Jonny Appleseed*, ch. 52.
15 Mistry, "Squatter," 315.
16 Choy, *All That Matters*, ch. 4.
17 Ibid.
18 Chariandy, *Brother*, 10.
19 Ibid.
20 Ibid, 46.
21 Ibid, 31.
22 Ibid, 16.
23 Ibid, 36.
24 Ibid, 39.
25 Ibid, 129.

26 Barrett, "Learning," 135.
27 Ondaatje, *English Patient*, 169–71.
28 Quoted in McMaster, "Sleep Is Like Sex."
29 Basile, "Sun, Moon, and Talia," 520.
30 Ondaatje, *English Patient*, 173, 257–8. The version of the story where Katharine does not speak is on pages 248–9.
31 Ibid., 5.
32 Ibid., 13.
33 Ibid., 103.
34 Fledderus, "English Patient," 48, 34.
35 Similar concerns arise in Ondaatje's *In the Skin of a Lion*, to which *The English Patient* is a quasi-sequel. *In the Skin of a Lion* also opens with Hana sacrificing her sleep for a man; she listens to her father's story while "she stays awake to keep him company" (1). Sleep also occurs in other intriguing forms in this novel, such as during the climactic scene where Patrick breaks into the water purification plant intending to blow it up but then falls asleep rather than detonating the bombs.
36 Abdou, *Bone Cage*, 83.
37 Lindberg, *Birdie*, 26.
38 Ibid., 18.
39 Mootoo, *Cereus Blooms*, 109, 120, 168.
40 Ricci, *Sleep*, 1.
41 On Ricci's personal experience, see Medley, "Author Nino Ricci."
42 I have drawn information on narcolepsy from reputable sources such as the Cleveland Clinic. Still, any misunderstandings are my own; do not take medical advice from an English professor, or from a novel for that matter. Unlike David, for example, many people with narcolepsy may find that their condition responds quite well to treatment.
43 Ricci, *Sleep*, 81.
44 Ibid., 82.
45 Ibid., 5.
46 Ibid., 167.
47 R.D. Cartwright, *Twenty-Four Hour Mind*, introduction.
48 Winter, *Sleep Solution*, 59.
49 Ricci, *Sleep*, 182.
50 Ibid., 75.
51 Dobson, "Shadow Sides."
52 Raso, dir., *Awake*.
53 Rotten Tomatoes, "Awake"; FlixPatrol, "Top Ten."
54 Orpana, *Gasoline Dreams*, 160.
55 Jameson, *Archaeologies of the Future*, 199.
56 Krasinski, dir., *A Quiet Place*.
57 Orpana, *Gasoline Dreams*, 29.

58 Daggett, *Birth of Energy*, 12.
59 M. Cartwright, "Pillow Book."
60 Buffam, *Pillow Book*, 3.
61 Ibid., 28.
62 Ibid., 20.
63 Ibid., 95.
64 Kondo, *Life-Changing Magic*, 190.
65 Buffam, *Pillow Book*, 15.
66 See, for example, ibid., 13.
67 Ibid., 17, 74, 74, 5.
68 Ibid., 47.
69 Montgomery, *Anne of Green Gables*, 120.
70 Schwenger, *At the Borders*, preface.
71 Balser, "*Marrow Thieves*."
72 Dimaline, *Marrow Thieves*, 53, 48.
73 Ibid., 88.
74 Ibid., 14.
75 Ibid., 29.
76 On the link between the medicalization of sleep and its commodification, see Arber, Meadows, and Venn, "Sleep and Society," 229–30.
77 Dimaline, *Marrow Thieves*, 2, 4.
78 As I discuss in the next chapter, scientists can now use MRI scans of sleeping people to read the general content of their dreams, an ability that is both exciting and frightening. Like so many dystopias, *The Marrow Thieves* is in some ways a little too real. Incidentally, Karen Russell's novella *Sleep Donation* has striking plot similarities to *The Marrow Thieves*. In Russell's dystopia, the population suffers from a terrible insomnia epidemic, and a corporation promises to extract the ability to sleep from those who still have it and to transfuse this ability into those who do not. In a disturbing turn, a baby proves to be the ideal donor. For a discussion of this book, see Reiss, *Wild Nights*, ch. 7.
79 Simpson, "Stories, Dreams, and Ceremonies."
80 Highway, "On Native Mythology," 24.
81 Ermine, "Aboriginal Epistemology," 108–9.
82 King, *Green Grass, Running Water*, 1.
83 Whyte, "Our Ancestors' Dystopia Now," 207.
84 Alongside the damage to Indigenous dreams in a conceptual sense, the effects of residential schools on those who were forced to attend often include literal insomnia and other symptoms of post-traumatic stress disorder, effects that are reflected in literary works such as Drew Hayden Taylor's *Motorcycles and Sweetgrass* and Tomson Highway's *Kiss of the Fur Queen*. See Song, "Residential School Experiences," 1580. Another striking representation of sleep as a site of power struggles in the context of residential schools occurs in Lee Maracle's story "Charlie."

85 Dimaline, *Marrow Thieves*, 65.
86 Ibid., 73.
87 Ibid., 74.
88 The architecture of this hotel also recalls Benjamin Reiss's comment that colonial authorities have a history of trying "to stamp out sleeping arrangements that they considered perverse." Reiss, *Wild Nights*, 25. The problem of colonization imposing norms that make Indigenous sleeping practices difficult is also taken up in Leanne Betasamosake Simpson's novel *Noopiming*, where some of the characters in colonized Ontario have trouble sleeping, but the practices that would help them to sleep, such as starting fires, are often prohibited.
89 Dimaline, *Marrow Thieves*, 139.
90 Ibid., 144.
91 Ibid.
92 Ibid., 172.
93 Ibid., 228.
94 Reiss, *Wild Nights*, 7.

INTERLUDE

1 For illuminating commentary on the loss of bedroom privacy in the pandemic, see Archer, "Myth of Bedroom Privacy."
2 North, "Pandemic Has Created."
3 Ibid.
4 See, for example, Robertson and Gebeloff, "How Millions of Women"; and Evelyn, "We're Expendable."
5 CBC *News*, "Pandemic Anxiety."
6 Renner, "Pandemic Is Giving People."
7 Ibid.
8 Cited in Weikle, "How to Keep."
9 Ibid.
10 Hamblin, "Mysterious Link."
11 North, "Pandemic Has Created."
12 See Tunney, "Court Grants Injunction." A photo by Justin Tang included in this article shows a counterprotestor holding a sign that says, "I Want Sleep."
13 Connley, "Why Many Employees."
14 Friedman, "Locked-Down Teens."
15 Rabson, "Half of COVID-19."
16 Hamblin, "Mysterious Link."
17 See, for example, Yates, "Fatigue after COVID."
18 BBC, "Story of Sleep."
19 Ibid.
20 BBC, "Max Richter's Sleep."
21 Snower, "Awakening."

22 Ibid.
23 *Daily Mail*, "Planes Sit Dormant."
24 Mandel, *Station Eleven*, 31.
25 Brand, "Dionne Brand."
26 C. Hall, "Canada's Not Trailing."
27 Quoted in Pinsker, "Year We Lost."
28 Mazda Canada, "Sleeping Roads."
29 My thanks to environmental humanities scholar Pamela Banting, who came up with the phrase "deficit of driving" upon hearing about the Mazda ad.
30 Marzovilla, "Skylar Grey."
31 Mazda is not the first automobile manufacturer to pitch its products as triumphant symbols of recovery from tragic social disruptions. During the late stages of the Second World War, after retooling its assembly lines to manufacture aircraft engines and tanks, Buick ran advertisements inviting soldiers to look forward to a new car purchase after the war. A Buick Roadmaster convertible with whitewall tires would be "so nice to come home to!" Nilsson, "Vintage Auto Ads."
32 Mazda Canada, "Together 15." The "Sleeping Roads" campaign also played on a Mazda ad from 2019, produced just a few months before the pandemic, called "Sleeping Cars." In this ad, viewers are reassured that because their Mazda 3 is available with all-wheel drive, they don't need to hide it under a tarp in a garage during icy winter months. The tagline reads, "The joy of driving should never sleep." Mazda Canada, "Sleeping Cars."
33 Williams, *Politics of Sleep*, introduction.
34 Heyes, "We're Not Dreamers."
35 K.S. Robinson, "Coronavirus."

CHAPTER FOUR

1 The reported number of times that average smartphone users check their phone varies depending on the year and the methodology. One study, for example, gives a figure of ninety-six phone checks per day. Cision, "Americans Check."
2 On this problem, see Crary, *24/7*, 13; and Hsu, "Sociological Significance," 870–1.
3 CBC *News*, "Teens Getting Less Sleep."
4 Reiss, *Wild Nights*, 206.
5 Greaney, *Sleep and the Novel*, ch. 6.
6 Walker, *Why We Sleep*, 325–7.
7 Ibid., 330, 339.
8 Joe Pinsker of the *Atlantic* notes that because the name Alexa is now associated so strongly with the subservience of Amazon's voice assistant, the number of parents giving the name Alexa to their babies has plummeted. For the well over 100,000 people already called Alexa in the United States alone, social life now poses new difficulties, such as intense bullying at school that has led parents to

change their child's name. The problem also causes more mundane frustrations; Pinsker cites a case where a father "asked his daughter Alexa for some water, and their robot Alexa responded by offering to order a case of Fiji water for $27." Pinsker, "Amazon Killed."

9 Costandi, "Brain Scans."

10 Working in the other direction, companies have also been experimenting with "targeted dream incubation," with Coors, for example, devising videos and soundscapes to generate "refreshing dreams" of Coors beer in their audience. See Gabbatt, "Nightmare Scenario."

11 Wajcman, "How Silicon Valley," 1272.

12 Ibid.

13 Ibid., 1285.

14 Ibid., 1286.

15 Ibid.

16 De Cristofaro and Chiodo, "Quantified Sleep," 176.

17 Ibid., 183.

18 Broussard, "Review."

19 Zraick and Mervosh, "That Sleep Tracker." On orthosomnia, see also De Cristofaro and Chiodo, "Quantified Sleep."

20 Duraccio et al., "Does iPhone Night Shift?"

21 Buckley, "Is Night Shift?"

22 Clover, "ios 14."

23 Stein, "How the Apple Watch."

24 Rossignol, "Apple Executives."

25 Reiss, *Wild Nights*, 204.

26 Bloomberg, "Workers Describe."

27 For discussion of this issue and related problems, see Birth, "While the West Sleeps," 121.

28 Crary, *24/7*, 3.

29 This 2021 figure comes from Polaris Market Research, "Sleeping Aids." Different methodologies, of course, provide different figures. In 2019, the mattress company Casper exuberantly estimated that the value of "the global Sleep Economy" was US$432 billion. Newman, "Is Casper's?"

30 Williams, *Politics of Sleep*, introduction.

31 The examples of defensive design given here are drawn from Pelley, "How 'Defensive Design'"; and Chellew, *#defensiveTO*.

32 Pelley, "How 'Defensive Design.'"

33 Wolf-Meyer, *Slumbering Masses*, 245.

34 Greaney, *Sleep and the Novel*, ch. 6.

35 Calm, "Calm."

36 Ibid.

37 LaVito, "Relaxation App Calm."

38 Battan, "Unsettling Anti-entertainment."

39 Unless otherwise indicated, dollar amounts are in Canadian currency.
40 Battan, "Unsettling Anti-entertainment."
41 Hartman, "Calm Is Sleeping."
42 Ibid.
43 Medem, "Once Upon a Time."
44 Interviewed in Smith, "Art of Writing."
45 Quoted in Purdon and Palleja, "Canada's Top 'Sleep Writer.'"
46 Ibid.
47 All the direct references to Sleep Stories in this section come from the Calm app. See Calm, "Calm."
48 Simon, creator, *The Wire*; Stahelski, dir. *John Wick*.
49 Woolf, *Mrs. Dalloway*, 3.
50 Quoted in Purdon and Palleja, "Canada's Top 'Sleep Writer.'"
51 Spielberg, dir., *Jurassic Park*.
52 Dray, "Jurassic World 3."
53 See, for example, Harrison, "Five Years."
54 See, for instance, Calm, "Meet the Writer."
55 Calm, "Welcome to Calm."
56 Mind Candy Ltd Moshi, "Moshi Twilight Sleep Stories."
57 Calm, "Introducing Calm Kids."
58 De Cristofaro and Chiodo, "Quantified Sleep," 178.
59 Rosa, *Social Acceleration*, 157.
60 Ibid., 128, original emphasis.
61 Abdou, *This One Wild Life*, 183.
62 Heyes, "Dead to the World," 370.
63 I am drawing here from the research of Lindsay Hahn cited in Gambini, "Media Use." Also of note is a peer-reviewed study of 10,000 Calm users, which found that "perceived improvement in falling asleep was positively associated with the use of Sleep Stories, sleep meditations and music/soundscapes." Huberty et al., "Can a Meditation App?" 7. The participants in this survey were Calm subscribers who had used the app recently, so to some extent they may have self-selected as being among those who find the app helpful.
64 De Cristofaro, "Counterproductive Promise."
65 Greaney, *Sleep and the Novel*, ch. 6.
66 Ibid.
67 Dewdney, *Acquainted with the Night*, 152.
68 Ibid., 152.
69 Ibid., 153.
70 Huber, *Assembling the Morrow*, 133.
71 Ibid., 7.
72 Ibid., 41.
73 Ibid., 22.
74 Ibid., 10.

75 Ibid.
76 Ibid., 24.
77 Ibid., 11.
78 Ibid., 12.
79 *Hamlet*, act 3, scene 1, line 66.
80 Huber, *Assembling the Morrow*, 13.
81 Ibid., 15.
82 Ibid., 17–18.
83 Ibid., 134.
84 Lorre and Prady, creators, "Anxiety Optimization."
85 Reitman, dir., *Ghostbusters*.
86 Huber, *Assembling the Morrow*, 135.
87 Ibid., 113.
88 Huber and Morse, "In Conversation."
89 Huber, *Assembling the Morrow*, 11.

CHAPTER FIVE

1 For details on the 2013 Alberta floods, see City of Calgary, "Flooding in Calgary"; and Davison and Powers, "Why Alberta's Floods." For information on how attribution studies can link climate change to specific weather events such as the 2013 floods and the 2021 heat dome, see Ness, "Are Extreme Weather Events?"
2 CBC *News*, "Calgary Mayor."
3 The information in this paragraph comes from Obradovich et al., "Nighttime Temperature." For a reader-friendly summary of the study, see Cross, "Scientists Warn."
4 On the Pakistan flood of 2022, see CBC *News*, "Pakistan's PM." On the drought in the Horn of Africa, see CBC *News*, "Deadly African Drought."
5 Lagos, Yemen, and Haiti belong to a list of places identified as most at risk of humanitarian crisis due to climate change. See Law, "Climate Crisis."
6 For the report indicating that Canada is warming twice as fast as the global average, see Environment and Climate Change Canada, "Canada's Climate." For comments on the "hundred-year floods" in Quebec, see Eschner, "Canada." Reporting on the fires of 2016 and 2023 is also widely available.
7 See Witze, "Racism Is Magnifying."
8 Halton, "Climate Change."
9 Uguen-Csenge and Lindsay, "For 3rd Straight Day."
10 Schmunk, "'Most Homes.'"
11 Canadian Institute for Climate Choices, *Health Costs*, 33. These numbers are based on the mid-range estimates for low- and high-emissions scenarios.
12 CBC *News*, "Coroner's Report"; Gomez, "June Heat Wave." Both articles note that most of the people who died were seniors. In global terms, Asia, India, and

eastern Europe have been suffering from the highest rates of heat-related excess deaths in this century. Zhao et al., "Global, Regional," fig. 2.

13 Schmunk, "In a Single Week."

14 CBC *News*, "2023 Wildfire Season."

15 Cited in Parmar and Doban, "BC Heatwave."

16 Ibid.

17 On insomnia and post-traumatic stress disorder in survivors of the Fort McMurray fire, see Purdy, "Fort McMurray Residents"; and Snowdon, "5 Years On."

18 Midnight Oil, "Beds Are Burning."

19 SBS *News*, "Midnight Oil."

20 Atwood, *Oryx and Crake*, 5.

21 Ibid., 5.

22 Ibid., 15.

23 Ibid., 337.

24 K.S. Robinson, *Ministry for the Future*, 1.

25 Ibid., 2.

26 Ibid., 12.

27 Ibid.

28 Ghosh, *Great Derangement*, 8. Some of my comments on Ghosh here are adapted from my review of Mockler et al., eds, *Watch Your Head*. Huebener, "Climate and Imagination."

29 Ghosh, *Great Derangement*, 72–3.

30 Vadnais, *Fauna*, 7.

31 Ibid., 28.

32 Ibid., 118.

33 Ibid., 119.

34 De Cristofaro, "Writing the Sleep Crisis."

35 Banting, "Suddenly." For an elaboration on the idea that the apocalypse has already occurred for Indigenous societies, see Whyte, "Our Ancestors' Dystopia Now," which I cite in chapter 3.

36 K.S. Robinson, *Ministry for the Future*, 4.

37 Lai, *Salt Fish Girl*, 85.

38 Ibid., 70.

39 See, for example, Zimmer, "Evolution of Sleep."

40 Borel, "Do Microbes Sleep?"

41 Discussion and notes on this topic are available in Freiberg, "Why We Sleep."

42 Wohlleben, *Hidden Life*, 142.

43 Yong, Lay, and Jimenez, "How the Animal."

44 Rattenborg, Lima, and Amlaner, "Facultative Control."

45 Yong, Lay, and Jimenez, "How the Animal."

46 Ortega, "Octopuses."

47 Hsu, "Sociological Significance," 867.
48 Ibid., 867–8.
49 Ibid., 869.
50 On seasonal sleep changes, see Clinton, "Humans 'May Need.'" On lunar phases, see Grover, "Lunar Cycle."
51 See Handley, "Two Four-Year Postdocs."
52 R. Sullivan, "Early Humans."
53 Rijo-Ferreira et al., "*Trypanosoma brucei.*"
54 Ibid. For wide-ranging commentary on what it means to live with circadian rhythms, see M. Hall, "Chronophilia."
55 Crary, *24/7*, 10.
56 Reiss, *Wild Nights*, 15.
57 Ibid., 15.
58 Mohamed, "Increase in LED Lighting."
59 For an explanation of the name of the Wiliideh, or Coney River, see Yellowknives Dene First Nation, "Our Land."
60 R. Wong, "sleepless," 89.
61 Hnatyshyn, "Decades of Arsenic."
62 Ibid. See also Strong, "Giant Mine."
63 Gleeson, "De Beers."
64 Ephron, dir., *Sleepless in Seattle*.
65 R. Wong, "what remains," 91.
66 Pound, "In a Station."
67 McKay, *Vis à Vis*, 27–8.
68 Ibid., 21.
69 Creates, *Sleeping Places, Newfoundland 1982*, 40.
70 McKay, *Deactivated West 100*, 17–18.
71 Macfarlane, "Hollow Places," 101.
72 Creates, "Marlene Creates," 13.
73 McKay, "Sleeping Places," 31–2. Also reprinted in Garvey and Kunard, eds, *Marlene Creates*, 48.
74 See Creates, *Dwelling and Transience*.
75 Szeman, "Foreword," vii.
76 Orpana, *Gasoline Dreams*, 47.
77 Ibid., 6. For information on carbon concentrations, see Kahn, "Earth's CO_2"; and Shulmeister, "Climate Explained."
78 Orpana, *Gasoline Dreams*, 51.
79 Ibid., 56.
80 Kubrick, dir., *2001: A Space Odyssey*.
81 Orpana, *Gasoline Dreams*, 66.
82 Preston, "Why Humans Sleep Less."
83 Orpana, *Gasoline Dreams*, 220.

CONCLUSION

1 Hale and Hale, "Is Justice Good?" 367, 365–6.
2 Jacobs, *Say Good Night*, xxvi.
3 North, "Pandemic Has Created."
4 Hamblin, "Mysterious Link."
5 Levine, *Geography of Time*, 141.
6 See, for example, Government of Canada, "New Realities."
7 Quoted in Velez, "Resting."
8 See, for example, my comments on Hersey's book in the introduction.

BIBLIOGRAPHY

Abdou, Angie. *The Bone Cage*. Edmonton: NeWest, 2007.

– *This One Wild Life: A Mother-Daughter Wilderness Memoir*. Toronto: ECW, 2021.

Amin, Mohammad M., Joseph Anthony Parisi, Morris S. Gold, and Avram R. Gold. "War-Related Illness Symptoms among Operation Iraqi Freedom/Operation Enduring Freedom Returnees." *Military Medicine* 175, no. 3 (2010): 155–7.

Arber, Sara, Robert Meadows, and Susan Venn. "Sleep and Society." In *The Oxford Handbook of Sleep and Sleep Disorders*, ed. Charles M. Morin and Colin A. Espie, 223–47. Oxford: Oxford University Press, 2012.

Archer, Sarah. "The Myth of Bedroom Privacy." *Vox*, 24 June 2021. https://www.vox.com/the-goods/22537487/bedroom-privacy-covid-work-from-home.

Arens, Rita, ed. *Sleep Is for the Weak: The Best of the Mommybloggers*. Chicago: Chicago Review, 2008.

"Arnold Schwarzenegger 2018 – The Speech That Broke the Internet – Most Inspiring Ever." YouTube, 2 May 2019. https://www.youtube.com/watch?v=u_ktRTWMX3M.

Athabasca University. "Mothers Who Don't Get Enough Sleep Age More Rapidly, Study Finds." 8 October 2021. https://news.athabascau.ca/faculty/faculty-of-humanities-social-sciences/new-mothers-who-dont-get-enough-sleep-age-more-rapidly-study-finds/.

Atwood, Margaret. *Oryx and Crake*. New York: Seal, 2003.

– "Variation on the Word *Sleep*." In *Selected Poems II: Poems Selected and New 1976–1986*, 77. Boston: Houghton Mifflin, 1987.

Aubrey, Allison. "Drug Ads Play Up Benefits, Downsize Risks." NPR, 13 April 2007. https://www.npr.org/templates/story/story.php?storyId=9571484.

Augustine. *The Confessions of Saint Augustine*. Trans. Edward B. Pusey. Christian Classics Ethereal Library. https://ccel.org/ccel/augustine/confess/.

Balser, Erin. "*The Marrow Thieves* by Cherie Dimaline Sells 100,000 Copies in Canada, Enters 20th Print Run." *CBC Books*, 5 February 2020. https://www.cbc.ca/books/the-marrow-thieves-by-cherie-dimaline-sells-100-000-copies-in-canada-1.5453205.

Banting, Pamela. "Suddenly." *NiCHE*, 17 January 2018. https://www.niche-canada.org/2018/01/17/suddenly.

Barnes, Adrian. *Nod*. London: Titan Books, 2015.

Barrett, Paul. "Learning to Memory Right." *Canadian Literature* 237 (2019): 134–5.

Basile, Giambattista. "Sun, Moon, and Talia." In *Il Pentamerone, Or the Tale of Tales*, vol. 2, trans. Richard Burton, 518–25. London: Henry and Company, 1893.

Battan, Carrie. "The Unsettling Anti-entertainment of 'A World of Calm.'" *New Yorker*, 27 October 2020. https://www.newyorker.com/culture/on-television/the-unsettling-anti-entertainment-of-a-world-of-calm.

BBC. "Max Richter's Sleep." https://www.bbc.co.uk/programmes/b06db5tv.

– "The Story of Sleep." https://www.bbc.co.uk/programmes/articles/2RgGQRZ27mV95jn8RZPWTM9/the-story-of-sleep.

Bell, Vaughan. "The Trippy State between Wakefulness and Sleep." *Atlantic*, 20 April 2016. https://www.theatlantic.com/science/archive/2016/04/deciphering-hypnagogia/478941/.

Belleau, Lesley. "Sunday at the Healing Lodge." In *An Anthology of Indigenous Literatures in English: Voices from Canada*, 5th ed., ed. Armand Garnet Ruffo and Katherena Vermette, 604–5. Oxford: Oxford University Press, 2020.

Berg, Maggie, and Barbara K. Seeber. *The Slow Professor: Challenging the Culture of Speed in the Academy*. Toronto: University of Toronto Press, 2016.

Bin, Yu Sun, Nathaniel S. Marshall, and Nick Glozier. "Sleeping at the Limits: The Changing Prevalence of Short and Long Sleep Durations in 10 Countries." *American Journal of Epidemiology* 177, no. 8 (2013): 826–33.

Birth, Kevin. "While the West Sleeps: Deglobed Globalization and Its Consequences." In *Time, Globalization and Human Experience*, ed. Paul Huebener, Susie O'Brien, Tony Porter, Liam Stockdale, and Yanqiu Rachel Zhou, 109–26. London: Routledge, 2017.

Bloomberg. "Workers Describe Harsh Conditions at Apple Supplier in China." *Chicago Tribune*, 16 January 2018. https://www.chicagotribune.com/business/blue-sky/ct-apple-china-workers-20180116-story.html.

Borel, Brooke. "Do Microbes Sleep?" *Popular Science*, 19 March 2014. https://www.popsci.com/blog-network/our-modern-plagues/do-microbes-sleep/.

Brand, Dionne. "Dionne Brand: On Narrative, Reckoning and the Calculus of Living and Dying." *Toronto Star*, 4 July 2020. https://www.thestar.com/entertainment/books/2020/07/04/dionne-brand-on-narrative-reckoning-and-the-calculus-of-living-and-dying.html.

– *In Another Place, Not Here*. New York: Grove, 1996.

– *Inventory*. Toronto: McClelland and Stewart, 2006.

– *Thirsty*. Toronto: McClelland and Stewart, 2002.

Broussard, Mitchel. "Review: Eight Sleep 'Pod Pro' iPhone-Connected Mattress Offers Temperature Controls and Sleep Tracking." *MacRumors*, 28 October 2020. https://www.macrumors.com/review/eight-sleep-pod-pro/.

Brown, Margaret Wise. *Goodnight Moon*. New York: Harper and Brothers, 1947.

Buckley, Cami. "Is Night Shift Really Helping You Sleep Better?" Brigham Young University, 25 April 2021. https://news.byu.edu/intellect/is-night-shift-really-helping-you-sleep-better.

Buffam, Suzanne. *A Pillow Book*. Toronto: Anansi, 2016.

Butler, Blake. *Nothing: A Portrait of Insomnia*. New York: Harper Perennial, 2011.

Butler, Jenna. *Magnetic North: Sea Voyage to Svalbard*. Kindle ed. Edmonton: University of Alberta Press, 2018.

Calhoun, Kenneth. *Black Moon*. New York: Penguin, 2014.

Calm. "Calm." App Store, Version 5.21. Accessed 5 July 2021. https://apps.apple.com/us/app/calm/id571800810.

– "The Coral City." *A World of Calm*, season 1, episode 1. HBO, 2020.

– "Introducing Calm Kids." 22 September 2021. https://www.calm.com/blog/introducing-calm-kids.

– "Meet the Writer behind the Sleep Story: Derrick Barnes." 12 February 2021. https://blog.calm.com/blog/meet-the-writer-behind-the-sleep-story-derrick-barnes.

– "Welcome to Calm." https://www.calm.com/blog/about.

Canadian Association of University Teachers. *Guide to Acknowledging First Peoples and Traditional Territory*. https://www.caut.ca/content/guide-acknowledging-first-peoples-traditional-territory.

Canadian Institute for Climate Choices. *The Health Costs of Climate Change: How Canada Can Adapt, Prepare, and Save Lives*. June 2021. https://climatechoices.ca/wp-content/uploads/2021/06/ClimateChoices_Health-report_Final_June2021.pdf.

Carson, Anne. "Every Exit Is an Entrance (A Praise of Sleep)." In *Decreation: Poetry, Essays, Opera*, 18–42. New York: Alfred A. Knopf, 2005.

Cartwright, Mark. "The Pillow Book." *World History Encyclopedia*, 20 April 2017. https://www.worldhistory.org/The_Pillow_Book/.

Cartwright, Rosalind D. *The Twenty-Four Hour Mind: The Role of Sleep and Dreaming in Our Emotional Lives*. Kindle ed. Oxford: Oxford University Press, 2010.

CBC. "Trudeau: 'There's No Place for the State in the Bedrooms of the Nation.'" Archive of original broadcast, 21 December 1967. https://www.cbc.ca/player/play/1260871747995.

CBC News. "Calgary Mayor to Flood Evacuees: 'Gather Your Valuables and Go.'" 20 June 2013. https://www.cbc.ca/news/canada/calgary/calgary-mayor-to-flood-evacuees-gather-your-valuables-and-go-1.1322031.

– "Coroner's Report on BC Heat-Dome Deaths Calls for Greater Support for Populations at Risk." 7 June 2022. https://www.cbc.ca/news/canada/british-columbia/bc-heat-dome-coroners-report-1.6480026.

– "Deadly African Drought Not Possible without Climate Change, Study Finds." 27 April 2023. https://www.cbc.ca/news/science/horn-of-africa-drought-climate-1.6824091.

– "New UVic Research into Physical Markers of Stress among Nurses Finds Disrupted Sleep Patterns." 30 January 2021. https://www.cbc.ca/news/canada/british-columbia/uvic-physiological-nursing-study-1.5894709.

– "Pakistan's PM Says Flood-Hit Areas Look 'Like a Sea.'" 7 September 2022. https://www.cbc.ca/news/world/pakistan-death-toll-passes-1300-1.6574417.
– "Pandemic Anxiety Causing Vivid Dreams, Expert Says." 22 April 2020. https://www.cbc.ca/news/canada/ottawa/pandemic-dreams-aiad-1.5540439.
– "Poor Quality, Short Sleep 'Prevalent' among Adults, StatsCan Says." 20 September 2017. https://www.cbc.ca/news/health/sleep-statistics-canada-1.4297378.
– "Teens Getting Less Sleep with Rise of Smartphones, Study Says." 3 November 2017. https://www.cbc.ca/news/health/teens-smartphones-sleep-decrease-1.4379024.
– "30% of Canadian Men Not Getting Enough Sleep, Says Study." 25 July 2016. https://www.cbc.ca/news/canada/british-columbia/lack-of-sleep-study-1.3693672.
– "The 2023 Wildfire Season Is Now BC's Most Destructive on Record – And It's Only Mid-July." 18 July 2023. https://www.cbc.ca/news/canada/british-columbia/bc-wildfire-july-18-1.6909596.
Centers for Disease Control and Prevention. "Sleep and Chronic Disease." 13 September 2022. https://www.cdc.gov/sleep/about_sleep/chronic_disease.html.
Centre for Sleep and Human Performance. "About." https://centreforsleep.com/about/about-us.html.
Chaput, Jean-Philippe, Suzy L. Wong, and Isabelle Michaud. "Duration and Quality of Sleep among Canadians Aged 18 to 79." Statistics Canada, 20 September 2017. https://www150.statcan.gc.ca/n1/pub/82-003-x/2017009/article/54857-eng.htm.
Chaput, Jean-Philippe, Jessica Yau, Deepa P. Rao, and Charles M. Morin. "Prevalence of Insomnia for Canadians Aged 6 to 79." Statistics Canada, 19 December 2018. https://www150.statcan.gc.ca/n1/pub/82-003-x/2018012/article/00002-eng.htm.
Chariandy, David. *Brother.* Toronto: McClelland and Stewart, 2017.
Chellew, Cara. *#defensiveTO*. https://www.defensiveto.com.
Choy, Wayson. *All That Matters*. ebook. Toronto: Anchor Canada, 2004.
Cision. "Americans Check Their Phones 96 Times a Day." 21 November 2019. https://www.prnewswire.com/news-releases/americans-check-their-phones-96-times-a-day-300962643.html.
City of Calgary. "Flooding in Calgary – Flood of 2013." https://www.calgary.ca/uep/water/flood-info/flooding-history-calgary.html.
Clark, Emily-Jane. *Sleep Is for the Weak: How to Survive When Your Baby Won't Go the F**k to Sleep*. London: Kyle Books, 2017.
Cleveland Clinic. "Here's What Happens When You Don't Get Enough Sleep (and How Much You Really Need a Night)." 25 March 2022. https://health.clevelandclinic.org/happens-body-dont-get-enough-sleep/.

Clinton, Jane. "Humans 'May Need More Sleep in Winter,' Study Finds." *Guardian*, 17 February 2023. https://www.theguardian.com/lifeandstyle/2023/feb/17/humans-may-need-more-sleep-in-winter-study-finds.

Clover, Juli. "IOS 14 and watchOS 7 Sleep Features: Sleep Mode, Wind Down, Sleep Tracking and More." *MacRumors*, 1 September 2020. https://www.macrumors.com/guide/sleep-tracking/.

Cohen, Leonard. "Two Went to Sleep." In *Parasites of Heaven*, 25. Toronto: McClelland and Stewart, 1966.

Connley, Courtney. "Why Many Employees Are Hoping to Work from Home Even after the Pandemic Is Over." CNBC *Make It*, 4 May 2020. https://www.cnbc.com/2020/05/04/why-many-employees-are-hoping-to-work-from-home-even-after-the-pandemic-is-over.html.

Cooper, Lydia R. "A Future Perfect: Queer Digital Sovereignty in Joshua Whitehead's *Jonny Appleseed* and *full-metal indigiqueer*." *Contemporary Literature* 60, no. 4 (2019): 491–514.

Costandi, Mo. "Brain Scans Decode Dream Content." *Guardian*, 5 April 2013. https://www.theguardian.com/science/neurophilosophy/2013/apr/05/brain-scans-decode-dream-content.

Crary, Jonathan. *24/7: Late Capitalism and the Ends of Sleep*. London: Verso, 2013.

Creates, Marlene. *Dwelling and Transience, Greater Victoria 2000*. Photo installation. 2000. http://www.marlenecreates.ca/works/2000dwelling.html.

– "Marlene Creates on Her Work." In *Marlene Creates: Places, Paths, and Pauses*, ed. Susan Gibson Garvey and Andrea Kunard, 13. Fredericton, NB: Goose Lane Editions and Beaverbrook Art Gallery, 2017.

– *Sleeping Places, Newfoundland 1982*. Photo installation. In *Marlene Creates: Places, Paths, and Pauses*, ed. Susan Gibson Garvey and Andrea Kunard, 40–7. Fredericton, NB: Goose Lane Editions and Beaverbrook Art Gallery, 2017.

Cross, Ryan. "Scientists Warn of Sleepless Nights in a Warming World." *Science*, 26 May 2017. https://www.sciencemag.org/news/2017/05/scientists-warn-sleepless-nights-warming-world.

CTV *News*. "Canada's First Napping Studio Offers Mid-day Snoozes for $10." 29 October 2019. https://www.ctvnews.ca/health/canada-s-first-napping-studio-offers-mid-day-snoozes-for-10-1.4661613.

Daggett, Cara New. *The Birth of Energy: Fossil Fuels, Thermodynamics, and the Politics of Work*. Durham, NC: Duke University Press, 2019.

Daily Hive. "Capture Photography Festival Billboards Covered Up after Intense Public Complaints." 7 April 2021. https://dailyhive.com/vancouver/capture-photography-festival-billboards-covered-steven-shearer.

Daily Mail. "Planes Sit Dormant as Airlines Struggle During Coronavirus." 19 May 2020. https://www.dailymail.co.uk/video/news/video-2157578/Video-Planes-sit-dormant-airlines-struggle-coronavirus.html.

Daschuk, James. *Clearing the Plains: Disease, Politics of Starvation, and the Loss of Indigenous Life*. New ed. Regina, SK: University of Regina Press, 2019.

Dater, Adrian. "Ambien Use for Insomnia Is Prevalent among NHL Players." *Denver Post*, 23 February 2013. https://www.denverpost.com/2013/02/23/ambien-use-for-insomnia-is-prevalent-among-nhl-players/.

Davison, Janet, and Lucas Powers. "Why Alberta's Floods Hit So Hard and Fast." CBC *News*, 22 June 2013. https://www.cbc.ca/news/canada/calgary/why-alberta-s-floods-hit-so-hard-and-fast-1.1328991.

De Cristofaro, Diletta. "The Counterproductive Promise of a 'Sleep Goal.'" *The Week*, 29 March 2022. https://theweek.com/tech/1011851/how-sleep-aids-ironically-devalue-sleep.

– "Writing the Sleep Crisis." *The Polyphony*, 11 December 2020. https://thepolyphony.org/2020/12/11/writing-the-sleep-crisis/.

De Cristofaro, Diletta, and Simona Chiodo. "Quantified Sleep: Self-Tracking Technologies and the Reshaping of 21st-Century Subjectivity." *Historical Social Research* 48, no. 2 (2023): 176–93.

Deerchild, Rosanna. "bread crumbs." In *An Anthology of Indigenous Literatures in English: Voices from Canada*, 5th ed., ed. Armand Garnet Ruffo and Katherena Vermette, 568–9. Oxford: Oxford University Press, 2020.

– "mama making moccasins." In *An Anthology of Indigenous Literatures in English: Voices from Canada*, 5th ed., ed. Armand Garnet Ruffo and Katherena Vermette, 565–6. Oxford: Oxford University Press, 2020.

dEMOTIONAL. "Sleep Is for the Weak." *State: In Denial*. Dead End Exit Records, 2013.

Devlin, Hannah. "Long Naps May Be Early Sign of Alzheimer's Disease, Study Shows." *Guardian*, 17 March 2022. https://www.theguardian.com/society/2022/mar/17/naps-early-sign-alzheimers-disease-study.

Dewdney, Christopher. *Acquainted with the Night: Excursions through the World after Dark*. Kindle ed. Toronto: HarperCollins, 2004.

Dimaline, Cherie. *The Marrow Thieves*. Toronto: DCB, 2017.

Dobson, Kit. "Shadow Sides." *Canadian Literature* 226 (2015): 157–9. https://canlit.ca/article/shadow-sides/.

Domanski, Don. "Hypnagogia." In *Fetishes of the Floating World*, 18–21. Kindle ed. Kingston, ON: Brick Books, 2021.

Donkin, Karissa. "Unsafe Sleep Practices Present in Hundreds of Infant Deaths in Canada, CBC Investigation Finds." CBC *News*, 3 May 2022. https://www.cbc.ca/news/canada/safe-sleep-investigation-1.6371261.

Dray, Kayleigh. "Jurassic World 3 Is Bringing Back Laura Dern's Ellie – aka the OG Film's Most Vital Character." *Stylist*, 2019. https://www.stylist.co.uk/long-reads/jurassic-park-ellie-sattler-laura-dern-feminist-hero-90s-kids-films-movies-dinosaurs/218543.

The Dreadnoughts. "Sleep Is for the Weak." *Polka's Not Dead*. Union Label Group, 2010.

Duraccio, Kara M., Kelsey K. Zaugg, Robyn C. Blackburn, and Chad D. Jensen. "Does iPhone Night Shift Mitigate Negative Effects of Smartphone Use on Sleep Outcomes in Emerging Adults?" *Sleep Health* 7, no. 4 (2021): 478–84.

Ekirch, A. Roger. *At Day's Close: Night in Times Past*. New York: W.W. Norton and Company, 2006.

Environment and Climate Change Canada. "Canada's Climate Is Warming Twice as Fast as Global Average." Government of Canada, 2 April 2019. https://www.canada.ca/en/environment-climate-change/news/2019/04/canadas-climate-is-warming-twice-as-fast-as-global-average.html.

Ephron, Nora, dir. *Sleepless in Seattle*. TriStar Pictures, 1993.

Ermine, Willie. "Aboriginal Epistemology." In *Introduction to Indigenous Literary Criticism in Canada*, ed. Heather Macfarlane and Armand Garnet Ruffo, 101–12. Peterborough, ON: Broadview, 2016.

Eschliman, Amy, and Leigh Oshirak. *Balance Is a Crock, Sleep Is for the Weak: An Indispensable Guide to Surviving Working Motherhood*. New York: Penguin, 2010.

Eschner, Kat. "Canada: Extreme Floods Show Climate Threat as Experts Warn of Further Tumult." *Guardian*, 30 April 2019. https://www.theguardian.com/world/2019/apr/30/canada-flooding-quebec-montreal-justin-trudeau-climate-change.

Evelyn, Kenya. "'We're Expendable': Black Americans Pay the Price as States Lift Lockdowns." *Guardian*, 25 May 2020. https://www.theguardian.com/world/2020/may/25/covid-19-lockdowns-african-americans-essential-workers.

Fagan, Brian. "The Bizarre Social History of Beds." *The Conversation*, 13 September 2019. https://theconversation.com/the-bizarre-social-history-of-beds-122517.

Findley, Timothy. *The Wars*. 1977. Reprint, Toronto: Penguin, 2014.

Fledderus, Bill. "'The English Patient Reposed in His Bed Like a [Fisher?] King': Elements of Grail Romance in Ondaatje's *The English Patient*." *Studies in Canadian Literature* 22, no. 1 (1997): 19–52.

FlixPatrol. "Top 10 on Netflix in the World on June 11, 2021." https://flixpatrol.com/top10/netflix/world/2021-06-11/.

Freiberg, Andrew S. "Why We Sleep: A Hypothesis for an Ultimate or Evolutionary Origin for Sleep and Other Physiological Rhythms." *Journal of Circadian Rhythms* 18, no. 2 (2020). https://www.ncbi.nlm.nih.gov/pmc/articles/PMC7120898/.

Friedman, Nicole. "Locked-Down Teens Stay Up All Night, Sleep All Day." *Wall Street Journal*, 22 May 2020. https://www.wsj.com/articles/locked-down-teens-stay-up-all-night-sleep-all-day-11590156291.

Gabbatt, Adam. "Nightmare Scenario: Alarm as Advertisers Seek to Plug into Our Dreams." *Guardian*, 5 July 2021. https://www.theguardian.com/media/2021/jul/05/advertisers-targeted-dream-incubation.

Gambini, Bert. "Media Use before Bed Can Be Beneficial." *UBNow*, 11 February 2022. https://www.buffalo.edu/ubnow/stories/2022/02/media-use-sleep.html.

Garvey, Susan Gibson, and Andrea Kunard, eds. *Marlene Creates: Places, Paths, and Pauses*. Fredericton, NB: Goose Lane Editions and Beaverbrook Art Gallery, 2017.

Ghosh, Amitav. *The Great Derangement: Climate Change and the Unthinkable.* Kindle ed. Chicago: University of Chicago Press, 2016.

Gleeson, Richard. "De Beers Gets Licence to Close Snap Lake Mine." CBC *News,* 22 May 2020. https://www.cbc.ca/news/canada/north/debeers-gets-licence-to-close-snap-lake-1.5581757.

Gomez, Michelle. "June Heat Wave Was the Deadliest Weather Event in Canadian History, Experts Say." CBC *News,* 2 October 2021. https://www.cbc.ca/news/canada/british-columbia/ubcm-heat-dome-panel-1.6189061.

Government of Canada. "The New Realities of Working Canadians: The Right to Disconnect and Gig Work Consultation." 17 May 2021. https://www.canada.ca/en/employment-social-development/corporate/portfolio/labour/programs/labour-standards/consultation-right-to-disconnect-and-gig-work.html.

Grandner, Michael A., Nirav P. Patel, Philip R. Gehrman, Dawei Xie, Daohang Sha, Terri Weaver, and Nalaka Gooneratne. "Who Gets the Best Sleep? Ethnic and Socioeconomic Factors Related to Sleep Complaints." *Sleep Medicine* 11, no. 5 (2010): 470–8.

Gray, Erin. "'The Good Sentences of Sleep': Parasomnia and 'Pataplay in Rawlings and Legris." *Open Letter* 13, no. 9 (2009): 153–65.

Greaney, Michael. *Sleep and the Novel: Fictions of Somnolence from Jane Austen to the Present.* ebook. London: Palgrave Macmillan, 2018.

Groeneveld, Sarah. "Unsettling the Environment: The Violence of Language in Angela Rawlings' *Wide Slumber for Lepidopterists.*" *ariel: a review of international english literature* 44, no. 4 (2013): 137–58.

Grover, Natalie. "Lunar Cycle Has Distinct Effect on Sleep, Study Suggests." *Guardian,* 27 January 2021. https://www.theguardian.com/lifeandstyle/2021/jan/27/lunar-cycle-has-distinct-effect-on-sleep-study-suggests.

Hale, Benjamin, and Lauren Hale. "Is Justice Good for Your Sleep? (And Therefore, Good For Your Health?)." *Social Theory and Health* 7, no. 4 (2009): 354–70.

Hall, Chris. "Canada's Not Trailing the World on Climate Action, Environment Minister Insists." CBC *Radio,* 24 April 2021. https://www.cbc.ca/radio/thehouse/jonathan-wilkinson-climate-carbon-trudeau-1.5999748.

Hall, Marcus. "Chronophilia; or, Biding Time in a Solar System." *Environmental Humanities* 11, no. 2 (2019): 373–401. https://read.dukeupress.edu/environmental-humanities/article/11/2/373/140791/Chronophilia-or-Biding-Time-in-a-Solar-System.

Halton, Mary. "Climate Change 'Impacts Women More Than Men.'" BBC *News,* 8 March 2018. https://www.bbc.com/news/science-environment-43294221.

Hamblin, James. "The Mysterious Link Between COVID-19 and Sleep." *Atlantic,* 21 December 2020. https://www.theatlantic.com/health/archive/2020/12/covid-19-sleep-pandemic-zzzz/617454/.

Handley, Sasha. "Two Four-Year Postdocs on the Environmental History of Sleep." *Environmental History Workshop,* 22 March 2021. https://

environmentalhistoryworkshop.wordpress.com/2021/03/22/two-four-year-postdocs-on-the-environmental-history-of-sleep/.

Harris, Gordon. "By Covering Up the Photographs of Steven Shearer, Vancouver Succumbed to Censorship." *Globe and Mail*, 24 April 2021. https://www.theglobeandmail.com/opinion/article-by-covering-up-the-photographs-of-steven-shearer-vancouver-succumbed/.

Harrison, Sara. "Five Years of Tech Diversity Reports – and Little Progress." *Wired*, 1 October 2019. https://www.wired.com/story/five-years-tech-diversity-reports-little-progress/.

Hartman, Liz. "Calm Is Sleeping Its Way to Success." *Publishers Weekly*, 16 August 2019. https://www.publishersweekly.com/pw/by-topic/digital/Apps/article/80952-calm-is-sleeping-its-way-to-success.html.

Haven Sleep Company. "Common Mattress Questions." https://havenmattress.ca/pages/haven-faq#reamaze#0#/kb/common-mattress-questions.

Heard, Catherine. "Vancouver Billboards by Artist Steven Shearer Evoked Intimacy Where People Least Expected It." *The Conversation*, 13 May 2021. https://theconversation.com/vancouver-billboards-by-artist-steven-shearer-evoked-intimacy-where-people-least-expected-it-160130.

Heckman-McKenna, Heather. "Redefining Love in Margaret Atwood's VARIATION ON THE WORD *SLEEP*." *Explicator* 74, no. 2 (2016): 92–8.

Hersey, Tricia. *Rest Is Resistance: A Manifesto*. New York: Little, Brown Spark, 2022.

Hertwig, Benjamin. "Home from the War." *Sun*, October 2017. https://www.thesunmagazine.org/issues/502/home-from-the-war.

– *Slow War*. Montreal and Kingston: McGill-Queen's University Press, 2017.

Heyes, Cressida J. "Anaesthetics of Existence." In *Feminist Phenomenology and Medicine*, ed. Kristin Zeiler and Lisa Folkmarson Käll, 263–84. Albany: State University of New York Press, 2014.

– "Dead to the World: Rape, Unconsciousness, and Social Media." *Signs: Journal of Women in Culture and Society* 41, no. 2 (2015): 361–83.

– "We're Not Dreamers, We're Doers: Sleep in the Neoliberal Imaginary." Public lecture presented by the interdisciplinary program in Gender Studies and the School of Culture and Communication, University of Melbourne, Parkville, Victoria, Australia, 7 December 2017.

Highway, Tomson. "On Native Mythology." In *Introduction to Indigenous Literary Criticism in Canada*, ed. Heather Macfarlane and Armand Garnet Ruffo, 21–4. Peterborough, ON: Broadview, 2016.

Hinds, Hilary. *A Cultural History of Twin Beds*. New York: Bloomsbury Academic, 2019.

Hnatyshyn, Olivia. "Decades of Arsenic Poisoning Produced by Giant Mine Has Caused Irreversible Damage to Dene First Nation Land." *Capital Current*, March 2021. https://capitalcurrent.ca/decades-of-arsenic-poisoning-produced-by-giant-mine-has-caused-irreversible-damage-to-yk-dene-first-nation-land/.

Holmes, Nancy. "'In Flanders Fields' – Canada's Official Poem: Breaking Faith." *Studies in Canadian Literature* 30, no. 1 (2005): 11–33.

Horne, Jim. *Sleeplessness: Assessing Sleep Need in Society Today*. Kindle ed. London: Palgrave Macmillan, 2016.

Hounsell, Kayla. "1 in 4 Seniors in New Brunswick Takes Sleeping Pills. A New Study Is Offering an Alternative." CBC *News*, 15 February 2021. https://www.cbc.ca/news/canada/nova-scotia/seniors-sleeping-pills-study-new-brunswick-1.5910922.

Hsu, Eric L. "The Sociological Significance of Non-human Sleep." *Sociology* 51, no. 4 (2017): 865–79.

Huber, Sandra. *Assembling the Morrow: A Poetics of Sleep*. Vancouver: Talonbooks, 2014.

Huber, Sandra, and Garry Thomas Morse. "In Conversation with Sandra Huber and Garry Thomas Morse." Talonbooks. https://talonbooks.com/meta-talon/in-conversation-with-sandra-huber-and-garry-thomas-morse.

Huberty, Jennifer, Megan E. Puzia, Linda Larkey, Ana-Maria Vranceanu, and Michael R. Irwin. "Can a Meditation App Help My Sleep? A Cross-Sectional Survey of Calm Users." PLOS *One* 16, no. 10 (2021). https://journals.plos.org/plosone/article?id=10.1371/journal.pone.0257518.

Huebener, Paul. "Climate and Imagination." Review essay on *Watch Your Head: Writers and Artists Respond to the Climate Crisis*, ed. Kathryn Mockler et al. *Canadian Literature* 251 (2022): 171–3. https://canlit.ca/article/climate-and-imagination/.

– *Nature's Broken Clocks: Reimagining Time in the Face of the Environmental Crisis*. Regina, SK: University of Regina Press, 2020.

Hufnagel, Jill. "Atwood's Variation on the Word Sleep." *Explicator* 54, no. 3 (1996): 188–91.

Ipellie, Alootook. "Waking Up." In *An Anthology of Indigenous Literatures in English: Voices from Canada*, 5th ed., ed. Armand Garnet Ruffo and Katherena Vermette, 293–6. Oxford: Oxford University Press, 2020.

Jacobs, Gregg D. *Say Good Night to Insomnia*. London: Henry Holt and Company, 2009.

Jameson, Fredric. *Archaeologies of the Future: The Desire Called Utopia and Other Science Fictions*. London: Verso, 2005.

Kahn, Brian. "Earth's CO_2 Passes the 400 PPM Threshold – Maybe Permanently." *Scientific American*, 27 September 2016. https://www.scientificamerican.com/article/earth-s-co2-passes-the-400-ppm-threshold-maybe-permanently/.

Kale, Sirin. "The Mattress Landfill Crisis: How the Race to Bring Us Better Beds Led to a Recycling Nightmare." *Guardian*, 12 February 2020. https://www.theguardian.com/environment/2020/feb/12/mattress-landfill-crisis-recycling-nightmare.

King, Thomas. *Green Grass, Running Water*. New York: Harper Perennial, 1993.

Kingsolver, Barbara. *Flight Behavior*. New York: Harper Perennial, 2012.

Kondo, Marie. *The Life-Changing Magic of Tidying Up: The Japanese Art of Decluttering and Organizing*. Trans. Cathy Hirano. Berkeley: Ten Speed, 2014.

Krasinski, John, dir. *A Quiet Place*. Paramount Pictures, 2018.

Kubrick, Stanley, dir. *2001: A Space Odyssey*. Metro-Goldwyn-Mayer, 1968.

Kulchyski, Peter. *Aboriginal Rights Are Not Human Rights: In Defence of Indigenous Struggles*. Winnipeg: ARP Books, 2013.

Lai, Larissa. *Salt Fish Girl*. Markham, ON: Thomas Allen, 2002.

Larsen, Karin. "Former Canucks Enforcer Tweets about 'Insane' Amount of Toradol and Ambien He Was Given in NHL." *CBC News*, 4 October 2021. https://www.cbc.ca/news/canada/british-columbia/former-canucks-enforcer-tweets-about-insane-amount-of-toradol-and-ambien-he-was-given-in-nhl-1.6199507.

LaVito, Angelica. "Relaxation App Calm Raises $88 Million, Valuing It $1 Billion." CNBC, 6 February 2019. https://www.cnbc.com/2019/02/05/calm-raises-88-million-valuing-the-meditation-app-at-1-billion.html.

Law, Tara. "The Climate Crisis Is Global, but These 6 Places Face the Most Severe Consequences." *Time*, 30 September 2019. https://time.com/5687470/cities-countries-most-affected-by-climate-change/.

Lee, Bruce Y. "Sleep Deprivation: Here's How Lack of Snooze Can Affect Your Walking, Balance." *Forbes*, 31 October 2021. https://www.forbes.com/sites/brucelee/2021/10/31/sleep-deprivation-heres-how-lack-of-snooze-can-affect-your-walking-balance/.

Legris, Sylvia. *Nerve Squall*. Toronto: Coach House Books, 2005.

Levine, Robert. *A Geography of Time: The Temporal Misadventures of a Social Psychologist, or How Every Culture Keeps Time Just a Little Bit Differently*. New York: Basic Books, 1997.

Lindberg, Tracey. *Birdie*. Toronto: HarperCollins, 2015.

Lockley, Steven W., and Russell G. Foster. *Sleep: A Very Short Introduction*. Oxford: Oxford University Press, 2012.

Lorre, Chuck, and Bill Prady, creators. "The Anxiety Optimization." *The Big Bang Theory*, season 8, episode 13. Warner Bros Television, 2015.

MacDonald, Gayle. "Canadians Are Not Getting Enough Sleep – And That's a Big Problem." *Globe and Mail*, 7 November 2022. https://www.theglobeandmail.com/life/style/article-sleep-crisis-canada/.

Macfarlane, Robert. "Hollow Places and Wordcaves." In *Marlene Creates: Places, Paths, and Pauses*, ed. Susan Gibson Garvey and Andrea Kunard, 101–6. Fredericton, NB: Goose Lane Editions and Beaverbrook Art Gallery, 2017.

Major, Alice. *Welcome to the Anthropocene*. Edmonton: University of Alberta Press, 2018.

Mandel, Emily St John. *Station Eleven*. Toronto: HarperCollins, 2014.

Maracle, Lee. "Charlie." In *An Anthology of Indigenous Literatures in English: Voices from Canada*, 5th ed., ed. Armand Garnet Ruffo and Katherena Vermette, 273–9. Oxford: Oxford University Press, 2020.

– *Daughters Are Forever*. Vancouver: Polestar, 2002.

Marsh, James H. "In Flanders Fields." *The Canadian Encyclopedia*, 24 February 2016. https://www.thecanadianencyclopedia.ca/en/article/in-flanders-fields.

Marzovilla, Julia. "Skylar Grey Helps Highlight 'A Good Cause on a Large Scale' with New Budweiser Super Bowl Commercial: Watch." *Billboard*, 26 January 2018. https://www.billboard.com/articles/news/super-bowl/8096489/skylar-grey-super-bowl-commercial-budweiser-stand-by-me.

Mayr, Suzette. *The Sleeping Car Porter*. Toronto: Coach House Books, 2022.

Mazda Canada. "Sleeping Cars." YouTube, 18 October 2019. https://www.youtube.com/watch?v=52UG3Ve_uAc.

– "Sleeping Roads." YouTube, 2 April 2020. https://www.youtube.com/watch?v=r5-3BtSLWtQ.

– "Together 15." YouTube, 20 May 2020. https://www.youtube.com/watch?v JYoE12WRDhA.

McAdam, Rhona. "The Hot Women." In *Ex-ville*, 25. Fernie: Oolichan Books, 2014.

McCrae, John. "In Flanders Fields." Reprinted in James H. Marsh, "In Flanders Fields," *The Canadian Encyclopedia*, 24 February 2016. https://www.thecanadianencyclopedia.ca/en/article/in-flanders-fields.

McCue, Duncan. "Lack of Sleep Is 'Epidemic' among Canadian Teens. Here's Why It Has Doctors Worried." *CBC News*, 29 January 2019. https://www.cbc.ca/news/health/national-sleep-deprivation-teenagers-youth-learning-1.4929842.

McCutcheon, Mark. "'Come on back to the war': Germany as the Other National Other in Canadian Popular Culture." *University of Toronto Quarterly* 78, no. 2 (2009): 764–81.

McGregor, Jonathan. "'Between history and a hard place': Benjamin Hertwig's *Slow War* and D.F. Brown's *Ghost of a Person Passing in Front of the Flag*." *War, Literature and the Arts: An International Journal of the Humanities* 30, nos 1–2 (2018). https://www.wlajournal.com/archives.

McKay, Don. *Deactivated West 100*. Kentville: Gaspereau, 2005.

– "Sleeping Places." In *Paradoxides*, 31–2. Toronto: McClelland and Stewart, 2012.

– *Vis à Vis: Field Notes on Poetry and Wilderness*. Kentville: Gaspereau, 2001.

McKinnon, Donna. "Feminist Philosopher and Political Theorist Cressida Heyes Named Henry Marshall Tory Chair." University of Alberta, 19 December 2018. https://www.ualberta.ca/arts/faculty-news/2018/december/feminist-philosopher-and-political-theorist-cressida-heyes-named-henry-marshall-tory-chair.html.

McMaster, Geoff. "Sleep Is Like Sex – We Aren't Getting Enough." *Folio*, 10 November 2016. https://www.folio.ca/sleep-is-like-sexwe-arent-getting-enough/.

Medem, María. "Once Upon a Time … Bedtime Stories Were Just for Kids." *New York Times*, 1 January 2022. https://www.nytimes.com/2022/01/01/style/bedtime-stories-for-adults.html.

Medley, Mark. "Author Nino Ricci Sheds Light on Life with Narcolepsy in New Thriller Novel." *Globe and Mail*, 18 September 2015. https://www.theglobeandmail.com/arts/books-and-media/author-nino-ricci-sheds-light-on-life-with-narcolepsy-in-new-thriller-novel/article26428380/.

Midnight Oil. "Beds Are Burning." *Diesel and Dust*. Columbia Records, 1987.

Mistry, Rohinton. "Squatter." In *The Harbrace Anthology of Short Fiction*, 5th ed., ed. Jon C. Stott and Raymond E. Jones, 300–17. Toronto: Nelson Education, 2012.

Mockler, Kathryn, et al., eds. *Watch Your Head: Writers and Artists Respond to the Climate Crisis*. Toronto: Coach House Books, 2020.

Mohamed, Waseem. "Increase in LED Lighting 'Risks Harming Human and Animal Health.'" *Guardian*, 14 September 2022. https://www.theguardian.com/environment/2022/sep/14/increase-in-led-lighting-risks-harming-human-and-animal-health.

Moncur, Bruce. "I Almost Died in the Afghanistan War, and for What?" *CBC News*, 17 August 2021. https://www.cbc.ca/news/canada/first-person-afghanistan-canadian-war-veteran-1.6142945.

Montgomery, Lucy Maud. *Anne of Green Gables*. 1908. Reprint, New York: Seal Books, 1996.

Moodie, Susanna. *Roughing It in the Bush*. 1852. Project Gutenberg, 16 March 2018. https://www.gutenberg.org/files/4389/4389-h/4389-h.htm.

Moore, Anna. "The Sexual Assault of Sleeping Women: The Hidden, Horrifying Rape Crisis in Our Bedrooms." *Guardian*, 15 June 2021. https://www.theguardian.com/society/2021/jun/15/the-sexual-assault-of-sleeping-women-the-hidden-horrifying-crisis-in-britains-bedrooms.

Mootoo, Shani. *Cereus Blooms at Night*. London: Granta Books, 1996.

Moshfegh, Ottessa. *My Year of Rest and Relaxation*. New York: Penguin, 2018.

Mind Candy Ltd Moshi. "Moshi Twilight Sleep Stories." https://apprecs.com/ios/1306719339/moshi-twilight-sleep-stories.

– "Sleep by Moshi." Facebook. Accessed 25 May 2020.

Nap It Up. "Services." http://napitup.ca/services/.

Ness, Ryan. "Are Extreme Weather Events the Result of Climate Change?" Canadian Climate Institute, 13 July 2021. https://climatechoices.ca/are-extreme-weather-events-the-result-of-climate-change/.

@netflix. "Sleep is my greatest enemy." *Twitter*, 17 April 2017, 5:32 p.m. https://www.twitter.com/netflix/status/854100194098520064.

Newman, Alex. "Is Casper's 'Sleep Economy' a Real Thing?" *Investing.com*, 3 March 2020. https://www.investing.com/analysis/is-caspers-sleep-economy-a-real-thing-200512658.

Nilsson, Jeff. "Vintage Auto Ads: Buick." *Saturday Evening Post*, 19 August 2015. https://www.saturdayeveningpost.com/2015/08/vintage-auto-ads-buick/.

Nobili, Lino, Luigi De Gennaro, Paola Proserpio, Fabio Moroni, Simone Sarasso, Andrea Pigorini, Fabrizio De Carli, and Michele Ferrara. "Local Aspects of

Sleep: Observations from Intracerebral Recordings in Humans." *Progress in Brain Research* 199 (2012): 219–32.

North, Anna. "The Pandemic Has Created a Nation of Insomniacs." *Vox*, 16 September 2021. https://www.vox.com/22671566/sleep-deprived-insomnia-covid-pandemic-stress-anxiety.

Nudelman, Franny. *Fighting Sleep: The War for the Mind and the US Military.* London: Verso, 2019.

Obradovich, Nick, Robyn Migliorini, Sara C. Mednick, and James H. Fowler. "Nighttime Temperature and Human Sleep Loss in a Changing Climate." *Science Advances* 3, no. 5 (2017): 1–6. https://www.science.org/doi/10.1126/sciadv.1601555.

Ondaatje, Michael. *The English Patient*. Toronto: Vintage Canada, 1992.

– *In the Skin of a Lion*. 1987. Reprint, Toronto: Vintage Canada, 1996.

The Onion. "Weighted Blanket Sure to Succeed Where CBD, Salt Lamp, Oil Diffuser, Acupressure Mat, Bath Bombs, and White Noise Machine Failed." 2 March 2020. https://www.theonion.com/weighted-blanket-sure-to-succeed-where-cbd-salt-lamp-1842015748.

Orpana, Simon. *Gasoline Dreams: Waking Up from Petroculture*. New York: Fordham University Press, 2021.

Ortega, Rodrigo Pérez. "Octopuses, Like Humans, Sleep in Two Stages." *Science*, 25 March 2021. https://www.science.org/content/article/octopuses-humans-sleep-two-stages.

Ortiz-Ospina, Esteban. "How Do People across the World Spend Their Time and What Does This Tell Us about Living Conditions?" *Our World in Data*, 8 December 2020. https://ourworldindata.org/time-use-living-conditions.

Parmar, Tarnjit, and Vanessa Doban. "BC Heatwave Causing Serious Sleep Struggles." *CityNews*, 29 June 2021. https://www.citynews1130.com/2021/06/27/bc-heat-wave-sleep/.

Patten, P.J. *Tower 25*. Vancouver: Cloudscape Comics, 2020.

Pelley, Lauren. "How 'Defensive Design' Leads to Rigid Benches, Metal Spikes, and 'Visual Violence' in Modern Cities." *CBC News*, 2 July 2019. https://www.cbc.ca/news/canada/toronto/how-defensive-design-leads-to-rigid-benches-metal-spikes-and-visual-violence-in-modern-cities-1.5192333.

Pinsker, Joe. "Amazon Killed the Name Alexa." *Atlantic*, 18 August 2021. https://www.theatlantic.com/family/archive/2021/08/amazon-alexa-popular-name/619794/.

– "The Year We Lost." *Atlantic*, 15 December 2020. https://www.theatlantic.com/family/archive/2020/12/2020-lost-year/617382/.

Polaris Market Research. "Sleeping Aids Market Share, Size, Trends, Industry Analysis Report, by Product (Mattresses & Pillows, Sleep Laboratories, Medications, Sleep Apnea Devices); by Sleep Disorders; by Region; Segment Forecast, 2022–2030." June 2022. https://www.polarismarketresearch.com/industry-analysis/sleeping-aids-market.

Pound, Ezra. "In a Station of the Metro." *Poetry* 2, no. 1 (1913): 12.

Preston, Elizabeth. "Why Humans Sleep Less Than Their Primate Relatives." *Smithsonian Magazine*, 6 May 2022. https://www.smithsonianmag.com/science-nature/why-humans-sleep-less-than-their-primate-relatives-180980018/.

Proust, Marcel. *In Search of Lost Time*. 7 vols. Trans. C.K. Scott Moncrieff (vols 1–6) and Sydney Schiff (vol. 7). 1927. Reprint, New York: Centaur Editions, 2016. https://archive.org/details/InSearchOfLostTimeCompleteVolumes/page/n1/mode/2up.

Purdon, Nick, and Leonardo Palleja. "Canada's Top 'Sleep Writer' Reveals How He Puts You Under (Can You Stay Awake?)." CBC *News*, 27 January 2019. https://www.cbc.ca/news/health/national-sleep-stories-chris-advansun-1.4929841.

Purdy, Chris. "Fort McMurray Residents Plagued by Sleepless Nights, Study Finds." *Toronto Star*, 16 August 2016. https://www.thestar.com/news/canada/2016/08/16/fort-mcmurray-residents-plagued-by-sleepless-nights-study-finds.html.

Rabson, Mia. "Half of COVID-19 Patients Report Symptoms after 12 Weeks, Health Agency Review Finds." CBC *News*, 7 July 2021. https://www.cbc.ca/news/politics/long-term-covid19-symptoms-phac-1.6093518.

Randall, David K. *Dreamland: Adventures in the Strange Science of Sleep*. New York: W.W. Norton and Company, 2012.

Rao, Gautam, Susan Redline, Frank Schilbach, Heather Schofield, and Mattie Toma. "Informing Sleep Policy through Field Experiments." *Science* 374, no. 6567 (2021): 530–3.

Raso, Mark, dir. *Awake*. Netflix, 2021.

Rattenborg, Niels C., Steven L. Lima, and Charles J. Amlaner, "Facultative Control of Avian Unihemispheric Sleep under the Risk of Predation." *Behavioural Brain Research* 105, no. 2 (1999): 163–72. https://www.sciencedirect.com/science/article/abs/pii/S0166432899000704.

rawlings, a. *Wide Slumber for Lepidopterists*. Toronto: Coach House Books, 2006.

Reiss, Benjamin. *Wild Nights: How Taming Sleep Created Our Restless World*. New York: Basic Books, 2017.

Reitman, Ivan, dir. *Ghostbusters*. Columbia Pictures, 1984.

Renner, Rebecca. "The Pandemic Is Giving People Vivid, Unusual Dreams. Here's Why." *National Geographic*, 15 April 2020. https://www.nationalgeographic.com/science/2020/04/coronavirus-pandemic-is-giving-people-vivid-unusual-dreams-here-is-why/.

Re:Searching for LGBTQ2S+ Health. "Two-Spirit Community." https://lgbtqhealth.ca/community/two-spirit.php.

Ricci, Nino. *Sleep*. Toronto: Anchor Canada, 2015.

Rich, Nathaniel. *Odds against Tomorrow*. New York: Farrar, Straus and Giroux, 2013.

Ricoeur, Paul. *Time and Narrative*. 3 vols. Trans. Kathleen McLaughlin and David Pellauer (vols 1–2) and Kathleen Blamey and David Pellauer (vol. 3). Chicago: University of Chicago Press, 1984–88.

Rijo-Ferreira, Filipa, Daniel Pinto-Neves, Nuno L. Barbosa-Morais, Joseph S. Takahashi, and Luisa M. Figueiredo. "*Trypanosoma brucei* Metabolism Is under Circadian Control." *Nature Microbiology*, 13 March 2017.

Robertson, Campbell, and Robert Gebeloff, "How Millions of Women Became the Most Essential Workers in America." *New York Times*, 18 April 2020. https://www.nytimes.com/2020/04/18/us/coronavirus-women-essential-workers.html.

Robinson, Eden. *Monkey Beach*. Toronto: Vintage Canada, 2000.

– *Son of a Trickster*. New York: Alfred A. Knopf, 2017.

Robinson, Kim Stanley. "The Coronavirus Is Rewriting Our Imaginations." *New Yorker*, 1 May 2020. https://www.newyorker.com/culture/annals-of-inquiry/the-coronavirus-and-our-future.

– *The Ministry for the Future*. Kindle ed. New York: Orbit, 2020.

Rosa, Hartmut. *Social Acceleration: A New Theory of Modernity*. Trans. Jonathan Trejo-Mathys. New York: Columbia University Press, 2013.

Rose, Janus. "Zuckerberg's Meta Endgame Is Monetizing All Human Behavior." *Vice*, 1 November 2021. https://www.vice.com/en/article/88g9vv/zuckerbergs-meta-endgame-is-monetizing-all-human-behavior.

Rossignol, Joe. "Apple Executives Discuss watchos 9's New Health Features Like AFib History and Tracking Your Sleep Stages." *MacRumors*, 13 June 2022. https://www.macrumors.com/2022/06/13/apple-watch-watchos-9-health-features/.

Ross-White, Amanda. "Sleeping on Your Back Increases Risks of Stillbirth." *The Conversation*, 12 October 2017. https://theconversation.com/sleeping-on-your-back-increases-risks-of-stillbirth-85236.

Rotten Tomatoes. "Awake." https://www.rottentomatoes.com/m/awake_2021.

Ruffo, Armand Garnet, and Katherena Vermette, eds. *An Anthology of Indigenous Literatures in English: Voices from Canada*. 5th ed. Oxford: Oxford University Press, 2020.

Russell, Karen. *Sleep Donation*. New York: Atavist Books, 2014.

SBS *News*. "Midnight Oil Song Joins Climate Change Fight." 3 September 2013. Accessed 1 November 2021. https://www.sbs.com.au/news/midnight-oil-song-joins-climate-change-fight.

Schmunk, Rhianna. "In a Single Week: A Timeline of How Once-in-a-Century Flooding Unfolded across BC." CBC *News*, 20 November 2021. https://newsinteractives.cbc.ca/longform/bc-flooding-2021-timeline-how-once-in-a-century-flooding-unfolded.

– "'Most Homes' in Lytton, BC, Destroyed by Catastrophic Fire, Minister Says." CBC *News*, 2 July 2021. https://www.cbc.ca/news/canada/british-columbia/bc-wildfires-lytton-july-1-2021-1.6087311.

Schwenger, Peter. *At the Borders of Sleep: On Liminal Literature*. Kindle ed. Minneapolis: University of Minnesota Press, 2012.

Scrivner, Lee. "That Sweet Secession: Sleep and Sleeplessness in Western Literature." In *Sleep: Multi-professional Perspectives*, ed. Andrew Green, Alex Westcombe, and Ved Varma, 268–90. Philadelphia: Jessica Kingsley, 2012.

Sharkey, Jackie. "Do Libraries Need Social Workers on Staff? Some Librarians Say Yes." CBC *News*, 16 March 2022. https://www.cbc.ca/news/canada/london/london-public-library-social-work-community-1.6386809.

Sharma, Sarah. *In the Meantime: Temporality and Cultural Politics*. Durham, NC: Duke University Press, 2014.

Shepherd, Kelly. "Crescent." In *Insomnia Bird: Edmonton Poems*, 92–3. Saskatoon, SK: Thistledown, 2018.

– "Cultural Darwinism for Dummies." In *Insomnia Bird: Edmonton Poems*, 26. Saskatoon, SK: Thistledown, 2018.

Shulmeister, James. "Climate Explained: What the World Was Like the Last Time Carbon Dioxide Levels Were at 400ppm." *The Conversation*, 7 July 2020. https://theconversation.com/climate-explained-what-the-world-was-like-the-last-time-carbon-dioxide-levels-were-at-400ppm-141784.

Simon, David, creator. *The Wire*. HBO, 2002–08.

Simpson, Leanne Betasamosake. *Noopiming: The Cure for White Ladies*. Toronto: Anansi, 2020.

– "Stories, Dreams, and Ceremonies: Anishinaabe Ways of Learning." *Tribal College: Journal of American Indian Higher Education* 11, no. 4 (2000). https://tribalcollegejournal.org/stories-dreams-ceremonies-anishinaabe-ways-learning/.

Sleep Country Canada. "About Us." https://www.sleepcountry.ca/about-us.

– "#SleepIsForTheStrong – Introducing Sleep Country's Bloom™ Mattress in a Box." YouTube, 5 June 2017. https://www.youtube.com/watch?v=2ghKbQQqBko.

– "Sleep Is the Fuel That Powers Your Day." Facebook, 11 July 2020.

– "Sleep Is the Fuel That Powers Your Day." Facebook, 17 July 2020.

– "To Power Your Day ... Start with a Good Night." Facebook, 14 July 2020.

– "Turn off the Lights. And Your Brain." YouTube, 27 September 2019. https://www.youtube.com/watch?v=6k-uTNwYf7s.

– "What Keeps You Awake?" YouTube, 11 February 2014. https://www.youtube.com/watch?v=6pOJ9driBVM.

Smith, Michael Acton. "The Art of Writing Sleep Stories." 27 April 2017. https://blog.calm.com/blog/the-thinking-behind-sleep-stories.

Snowdon, Wallis. "5 Years On, Psychological Wounds of Fort McMurray Wildfire Inflamed by New Trauma." CBC *News*, 3 May 2021. https://www.cbc.ca/news/canada/edmonton/fort-mcmurray-wildfire-anniversary-mental-health-1.6009169.

Snower, Dennis J. "Awakening in the Post-pandemic World." Brookings Institution, 27 March 2020. https://www.brookings.edu/blog/future-development/2020/03/27/awakening-in-the-post-pandemic-world/.

Song, Chengcheng. "The Residential School Experiences in Drew Hayden Taylor's *Motorcycles & Sweetgrass* and Tomson Highway's *Kiss of the Fur Queen*." *Theory and Practice in Language Studies* 8, no. 12 (2018): 1575–81.

Spielberg, Steven, dir. *Jurassic Park*. Universal Pictures, 1993.

Stahelski, Chad, dir. *John Wick*. Summit Entertainment, 2014.

Statistics Canada. "Table 45-10-0014-01: Daily Average Time Spent in Hours on Various Activities by Age Group and Sex, 15 Years and Over, Canada and Provinces." 3 April 2019. https://www150.statcan.gc.ca/t1/tbl1/en/tv.action?pid=4510001401.

Stein, Scott. "How the Apple Watch Tracks Sleep – And Why." CNET, 29 June 2020. https://www.cnet.com/health/sleep/how-the-apple-watch-tracks-sleep-and-why/.

Stern, Carly. "The College Mantra: Sleep Is For The Weak." *HuffPost*, 30 March 2016. https://www.huffpost.com/entry/college-mantra-sleep-for-the-weak_b_9557654.

Strong, Walter. "Giant Mine Arsenic Could Be Cleaned Up in 5 Years, Researcher Says." CBC *News*, 26 November 2017. https://www.cbc.ca/news/canada/north/giant-mine-arsenic-process-1.4418862.

Sugars, Cynthia. *Canadian Gothic: Literature, History, and the Spectre of Self-Invention*. ebook. Cardiff: University of Wales Press, 2014.

Sullivan, Garrett A., Jr. *Sleep, Romance and Human Embodiment: Vitality from Spenser to Milton*. Cambridge, UK: Cambridge University Press, 2012.

Sullivan, Rory. "Early Humans May Have Hibernated to Weather Harsh Winters, Say Researchers." *Independent*, 20 December 2020. https://www.independent.co.uk/news/science/archaeology/early-humans-hibernation-winter-atapuerca-spain-b1776824.html.

Szeman, Imre. "Foreword." In Simon Orpana, *Gasoline Dreams: Waking Up from Petroculture*, vii–xi. New York: Fordham University Press, 2021.

Thompson, Derek. "Can Medieval Sleeping Habits Fix America's Insomnia?" *Atlantic*, 27 January 2022. https://www.theatlantic.com/ideas/archive/2022/01/medieval-sleeping-habits-insomnia-segmented-biphasic/621372/.

Traill, Catharine Parr. *The Backwoods of Canada*. 1836. Project Gutenberg, 4 August 2013. https://www.gutenberg.org/ebooks/13559.

Tunney, Catharine. "Court Grants Injunction to Silence Honking in Downtown Ottawa for 10 Days." CBC *News*, 7 February 2022. https://www.cbc.ca/news/politics/injunction-ottawa-granted-1.6342468.

Turner, Logan. "Images of Security, City Staff Photographing 2 Men Sleeping on Thunder Bay, Ont., Bench Spark Outrage." CBC *News*, 23 April 2021. https://www.cbc.ca/news/canada/thunder-bay/tbay-transit-photos-spark-outrage-1.6000018.

Uguen-Csenge, Eva, and Bethany Lindsay. "For 3rd Straight Day, BC Village Smashes Record for Highest Canadian Temperature at 49.6 C." *CBC News*, 30 June 2021. https://www.cbc.ca/news/canada/british-columbia/bc-alberta-heat-wave-heat-dome-temperature-records-1.6084203.

Vadnais, Christiane. *Fauna*. Trans. Pablo Strauss. Kindle ed. Toronto: Coach House Books, 2020.

Velez, Brontë. "Resting on and for the Earth." *Atmos*, 28 April 2021. https://atmos.earth/rest-resistance-colonization-black-liberation/.

Villegas, Paloma E. "'I can't even buy a bed because I don't know if I'll have to leave tomorrow': Temporal Orientations among Mexican Precarious Status Migrants in Toronto." *Citizenship Studies* 18, nos 3–4 (2014): 277–91.

Vizenor, Gerald. *Manifest Manners: Narratives on Postindian Survivance*. Lincoln: University of Nebraska Press, 1994.

Wajcman, Judy. "How Silicon Valley Sets Time." *New Media and Society* 21, no. 6 (2019): 1272–89.

Walker, Karen Thompson. *The Dreamers*. New York: Penguin, 2019.

Walker, Matthew. *Why We Sleep: Unlocking the Power of Sleep and Dreams*. New York: Scribner, 2017.

Wall, Emmy Lee. "Statement on Removal of Arbutus Greenway Billboards." *Capture Photography Festival*, 6 April 2021. https://capturephotofest.com/statement-on-the-removal-of-the-arbutus-greenway-billboards/.

Wang, Chinchin, Rachel C. Colley, Karen C. Roberts, Jean-Philippe Chaput, and Wendy Thompson. "Sleep Behaviours among Canadian Adults: Findings from the 2020 Canadian Community Health Survey Healthy Living Rapid Response Module." Statistics Canada, 16 March 2022. https://www150.statcan.gc.ca/n1/pub/82-003-x/2022003/article/00001-eng.htm.

Waterfield, Geoff. "Strong Rebuke from Union at Social Media." *Country 105*, 25 April 2021. https://www.country1053.ca/2021/04/25/strong-rebuke-from-union-at-social-media/.

Watt-Cloutier, Sheila. *The Right to Be Cold: One Woman's Story of Protecting Her Culture, the Arctic, and the Whole Planet*. ebook. London: Allen Lane, 2015.

Weikle, Brandie. "How to Keep COVID-19 Stress from Ruining Your Sleep." *CBC News*, 5 April 2020. www.cbc.ca/news/health/covid-19-insomnia-1.5521402.

Whitehead, Joshua. *Jonny Appleseed*. ebook. Vancouver: Arsenal Pulp, 2018.

Whyte, Kyle Powys. "Indigenous Climate Change Studies: Indigenizing Futures, Decolonizing the Anthropocene." *English Language Notes* 55, nos 1–2 (2017): 153–62.

– "Our Ancestors' Dystopia Now: Indigenous Conservation and the Anthropocene." In *The Routledge Companion to the Environmental Humanities*, ed. Ursula K. Heise, Jon Christensen, and Michelle Niemann, 206–15. London: Routledge, 2017.

Wible, Pamela. "What I've Learned from My Tally of 757 Doctor Suicides." *Washington Post*, 13 January 2018. https://www.washingtonpost.com/national/

health-science/what-ive-learned-from-my-tally-of-757-doctor-suicides/2018/01/12/b0ea9126-eb50-11e7-9f92-10a2203f6c8d_story.html.

Williams, Simon J. *The Politics of Sleep: Governing (Un)consciousness in the Late Modern Age*. Kindle ed. London: Palgrave Macmillan, 2011.

Winter, W. Chris. *The Sleep Solution: Why Your Sleep Is Broken and How to Fix It*. New York: Berkley, 2017.

Witze, Alexandra. "Racism Is Magnifying the Deadly Impact of Rising City Heat." *Nature*, 14 July 2021. https://www.nature.com/articles/d41586-021-01881-4.

Wohlleben, Peter. *The Hidden Life of Trees: What They Feel, How They Communicate*. Vancouver: Greystone Books, 2015.

Wolf-Meyer, Matthew J. *The Slumbering Masses: Sleep, Medicine, and Modern American Life*. Kindle ed. Minneapolis: University of Minnesota Press, 2012.

Wong, Rita. "sleepless in Somba K'e." In *undercurrent*, 89–90. Gibsons, BC: Nightwood Editions, 2015.

– "what remains." In *undercurrent*, 91–2. Gibsons, BC: Nightwood Editions, 2015.

Wong, Teresa. *Dear Scarlet: The Story of My Postpartum Depression*. Vancouver: Arsenal Pulp, 2019.

Woolf, Virginia. *Mrs. Dalloway*. San Diego: Harcourt, 1925.

Worthman, Carol M. "Developmental Cultural Ecology of Sleep." In *Sleep and Development: Familial and Socio-cultural Considerations*, ed. Mona El-Sheikh, 167–94. Oxford: Oxford University Press, 2011.

Yates, Natasha. "Fatigue after COVID Is Way More Than Just Feeling Tired. 5 Tips on What to Do about It." *The Conversation*, 6 April 2022. https://theconversation.com/fatigue-after-covid-is-way-more-than-just-feeling-tired-5-tips-on-what-to-do-about-it-179478.

Yellowknives Dene First Nation. "Our Land." https://web.archive.org/web/20220815014953/https://ykdene.com/about/our-land/.

Yong, Ed, Jackie Lay, and Brian Jimenez. "How the Animal Kingdom Sleeps." *Atlantic*, 28 December 2017. https://www.theatlantic.com/video/index/549035/how-animals-sleep/.

Younging, Gregory. *Elements of Indigenous Style: A Guide for Writing by and about Indigenous Peoples*. Edmonton: Brush Education, 2018.

Yousef, Tareq. "There's No Evidence That Blue-Light Blocking Glasses Help with Sleep." *The Conversation*, 7 September 2020. https://theconversation.com/theres-no-evidence-that-blue-light-blocking-glasses-help-with-sleep-143523.

Zhao, Qi, Yuming Guo, Tingting Ye, Antonio Gasparrini, Shilu Tong, Ala Overcenco, Aleš Urban, et al. "Global, Regional, and National Burden of Mortality Associated with Non-optimal Ambient Temperatures from 2000 to 2019: A Three-Stage Modelling Study." *Lancet Planetary Health* 5, no. 7 (2021). https://www.thelancet.com/journals/lanplh/article/PIIS2542-5196(21)00081-4/fulltext.

Zhou, Yanqiu Rachel, and Kelly Coxson. "'Resilient' Social Workers: A New Spirit in Human Services, or a New Form of Governmentality?" In *Reworking*

Resilience, ed. Paul Huebener, Susie O'Brien, Tony Porter, Liam Stockdale, and Y. Rachel Zhou, 62–6. Hamilton, ON: Institute on Globalization and the Human Condition, McMaster University, 2017. https://globalization.socsci.mcmaster.ca/documents/ighc-working-paper-series_17_1_reworking-resilience.pdf.

Zimmer, Carl. "The Evolution of Sleep: 700 Million Years of Melatonin." *New York Times*, 2 October 2014. https://www.nytimes.com/2014/10/02/science/the-evolution-of-sleep-700-million-years-of-melatonin.html.

Zraick, Karen, and Sarah Mervosh. "That Sleep Tracker Could Make Your Insomnia Worse." *New York Times*, 13 June 2019. https://www.nytimes.com/2019/06/13/health/sleep-tracker-insomnia-orthosomnia.html.

INDEX

Page numbers in italics indicate references to figures.